Emergency Ultrasound

PRINCIPLES AND PRACTICE

Emergency Ultrasound
PRINCIPLES AND PRACTICE

Romolo Joseph Gaspari, M.D., M.Sc., R.D.M.S.
Assistant Professor of Emergency Medicine
Director, Division of Emergency Ultrasound
Department of Emergency Medicine
University of Massachusetts School of Medicine
Worcester, Massachusetts

J. Christian Fox, M.D., R.D.M.S.
Assistant Clinical Professor of Emergency Medicine
Director of Emergency Ultrasound
Department of Emergency Medicine
University of California
Irvine Medical Center
Orange, California

Paul R. Sierzenski, M.D., R.D.M.S.
President, Emergency Ultrasound Consultants
LLC Director, Emergency Ultrasound Fellowship
Program Director, Emergency and Trauma Ultrasound
Department of Emergency Medicine
Christiana Care Health System
Newark, Delaware

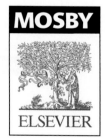

MOSBY

ELSEVIER

MOSBY
ELSEVIER

1600 John F. Kennedy Blvd.
Suite 1800
Philadelphia, Pennsylvania 19103-2899

EMERGENCY ULTRASOUND: PRINCIPLES AND PRACTICE   ISBN-13: 978-0-323-03750-1
Copyright 2006 by Mosby, Inc. All rights reserved.   ISBN-10: 0-323-03750-X

Library of Congress Cataloging-in-Publication Data

Gaspari, Romolo Joseph.
  Emergency ultrasound/Romolo Joseph Gaspari, J. Christian Fox,
Paul R. Sierzenski.–1st ed.
    p.cm.
  ISBN 0-323-03750-X
    1. Diagnosis, Ultrasonic, 2. Emergency medicine—Diagnosis. I. Fox,
J. Christian. II. Sierzenski, Paul R. III. Title.

  RC78.7.U4G37 2006
  616.07'543—dc22

                                2005041636

Acquisitions Editor: *Todd Hummel*
Editorial Assistant: *Martha Limbach*

Printed in China.

Last digit is the print number: 9 8 7 6 5 4 3 2 1

PREFACE

Emergency ultrasound is the offshoot of an imaging modality that has its roots in the specialty of radiology. Over time, ultrasound has migrated to a wide range of clinical practices such as obstetrics, cardiology, and vascular surgery. In the last decade, pioneers in emergency medicine have advanced the field of emergency ultrasound. From the first lonely fellowship, emergency ultrasound has evolved into a recognized core skill of graduating emergency residents. For a few of us, ultrasound has become integral to the practice of emergency medicine, and for others a useful adjunct in a busy emergency department.

Over the next decade I expect we will see an explosion of ultrasound in the emergency department, intensive care unit, and primary care offices. This book will direct clinical sonographers in the common focused ultrasound protocols encountered in the emergency department, ICU, and clinic. This book was written by practicing emergency physician sonographers for physicians who are integrating emergency ultrasound into their clinical practice. It is a practical reference on how to acquire the images needed to perform a focused ultrasound.

I am indebted to the initial ultrasound fellows and fellowship directors for their pioneering work that has made this book possible.

Romolo Gaspari

CONTENTS

INTRODUCTION AND BASICS

Introduction to Emergency Ultrasound

1

Romolo Gaspari and Paul Sierzenski

OVERVIEW

The goal of this book is to provide information and an approach on how to obtain, document, and integrate emergency ultrasound into your clinical practice. Specifically, we will show

- Standardization of image documentation for both still images and video images
- Tutorial on how ultrasound probe acquires images and how movement of the probe affects images seen on the ultrasound screen
- Step-by-step information on how to obtain ultrasound images
- Description of protocols for bedside ultrasound that answer routinely encountered clinical questions seen in emergent conditions
- Examples of normal ultrasound images
- Simplified drawings of all ultrasound images
- Diagrammatic representation of ultrasound scanning planes
- Examples of commonly encountered alternative ultrasound views resulting from unusual probe placement

BOOK ORGANIZATION

Each chapter is organized to provide instruction on how to successfully integrate bedside ultrasound into clinical practice. Chapter sections include

- Goal of protocol
- General anatomy
- Patient positioning
- Equipment
- Key ultrasound images
  - Landmarks
  - Image elements
  - Tricks of the trade
  - Partial view ultrasound images
- Alternative ultrasound images
- Ultrasound protocol techniques

ULTRASOUND IMAGE DRAWINGS

Ultrasound image drawings accompany each description.
- Simplified drawings showing only pertinent anatomy
- Unified color-coded anatomic drawings and ultrasound sector drawings
- Identification of common ultrasound artifacts

DEFINITIONS

In General

- **Protocol** – series of ultrasound views that answer a clinical question or that interrogate an organ or organ system
- **Image elements** – portions of ultrasound images corresponding to anatomic or pathologic structures within body
- **Partial view ultrasound images** – atypical or unusual ultrasound images that may contain some image elements needed for patient care but are missing crucial elements needed to complete ultrasound

Directions or Probe Movements

- **Cephalad** or **superior** – toward the head
- **Caudad** or **inferior** – toward the feet
- **Deep** or **posterior** – further from the anterior skin surface
- **Shallow** or **anterior** – closer to the anterior skin surface
- **Sliding** – moving probe parallel to probe indicator
- **Fanning** – moving probe perpendicular to indicator
- **Rotating** – turning probe in clockwise or counter-clockwise manner without moving probe on skin surface

Descriptive Terms

- **Hyperechoic** – increased brightness of a portion of ultrasound image (image is whiter)
- **Hypoechoic** – decreased brightness of a portion of ultrasound image (image is darker)
- **Anechoic** – lack of ultrasound echoes in a portion of ultrasound image (image is black)
- **Isoechoic** – similar echo levels as surrounding images
- **Heterogeneous** – uneven echo pattern within portion of ultrasound image
- **Homogeneous** – even echo pattern within portion of ultrasound image
- **Cystic** – anechoic structure with rounded edges

HOW TO THIS USE BOOK

Each chapter provides step-by-step instructions on how to accurately acquire and record all ultrasound images needed to answer clinical questions.

Anatomy

- Drawings and descriptions to help identify and visualize anatomy in two and three dimensions
  - Two dimensions – anatomy as drawn on paper or seen on screen
  - Three dimensions – anatomy as encountered during ultrasound procedure
- Understand how ultrasound probe movements affect imaging
      (Note: Only limited anatomy is depicted in this book. Additional textbooks on anatomy are required prior to using this book.)

Patient Positioning

• Identify proper patient positioning for obtaining ultrasound images

Equipment

• Proper probe selection for obtaining ultrasound images

Ultrasound Images

• Locate and identify anatomy needed to accurately frame ultrasound image
• Identify image elements where typical pathologic findings are located (where to look on ultrasound image to find typical pathology)
• Tricks of the trade to help avoid common pitfalls

Partial View Probe Positioning

• Suboptimal images that must be combined with other partial view images to complete an ultrasound protocol
• Multiple partial views required in some patients to complete protocol
• Drawings and labels corresponding to partial view images
• Allows identification of suboptimal views and identification of missing image components

Ultrasound Protocol

• Identify probe location, orientation, and probe movements for obtaining ultrasound images
• Identify ultrasound planes of imaging for obtaining ultrasound images
• Identify still image sequence or videotape images required for documenting lack of pathology

CONCEPT OF EMERGENCY ULTRASOUND

• Performance of ultrasound imaging by clinicians directly involved in patient care or sonographers working closely with medical staff
• Acquisition of images, interpretation of images, and integration into patient care performed by single individual
• Limited protocols focusing on questions common to emergent conditions
• Image acquisition occurs at site of patient care (bedside imaging)
• Focuses on yes–no questions important to emergent conditions
• Immediate integration of image interpretation with history, physical exam, laboratory, or additional imaging findings
• Non-protocol–driven ultrasound to assist in procedures performed by the clinician

ISSUES IN EMERGENCY ULTRASOUND

• Performing an ultrasound should not delay performing potential life-saving procedures
    Example: Holding a patient in the emergency department solely to perform a FAST (focused assessment sonography of trauma) exam when vital signs are rapidly deteriorating
• Repeat ultrasounds may be appropriate when patient condition changes
• In many emergent situations lack of patient prep (i.e., fasting, bladder filling) may result in decreased image quality or inability to obtain interpretable images

- In some situations, especially when first beginning to use ultrasound, the technology performs better to include a pathologic state (positive predictive value) rather than exclude it (negative predictive value) (e.g., it is easier to identify epididymitis than to exclude testicular torsion)
- In some emergent situations the usual ultrasound windows (place on body to put probe) are not accessible and alternative views must be used
    Example: It may be difficult to obtain a parasternal long cardiac view in a person with a pneumothorax

PATIENT DISCLOSURES

- When initiating an emergency ultrasound during your training phase, inform the patient that you may need to re-image the object of interest with additional imaging [e.g., a stable patient with a positive FAST may get a CAT (computerized axial tomography) scan or a patient with a limited ultrasound of the heart may get an echocardiogram by cardiology]
- Avoid using the terms "formal," "real," or "better" as a descriptor of later ultrasounds performed by radiology, cardiology, or OB/GYN. Use the term "confirmatory" or "consultation" (e.g., "Mrs. Jones I was not able to obtain the information I need to help treat you. I need to send you to radiology for additional confirmatory studies").
- Avoid using common descriptors such as "normal" or "okay"; this may be interpreted by the patient beyond what you intend. Describe for the patient *only* the yes–no question you are trying to answer (e.g., do not say the heart looks "normal"; instead tell the patient there is "no pericardial effusion, or fluid, around the heart." Do not say the baby looks "okay"; instead say there is a "pregnancy within the uterus with a heart beat").
- Do not provide patients with still images unless this is agreed upon with other consultants for follow-up

GENERAL CONCEPTS OF ULTRASOUND IMAGING

- Practice obtaining ultrasounds that match images in this textbook
- Practice identifying normal anatomy in ultrasound images
- Practice optimizing image quality by maximizing machine controls
- Fill screen area with objects of interest

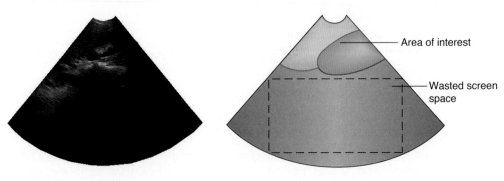

Depth set too deep

- Center area of interest in middle of screen

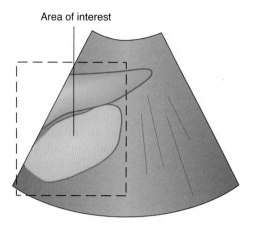

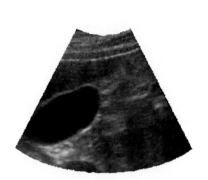

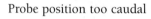

Probe position too caudal

- Any anatomic structure of interest should be imaged in at least two planes that are perpendicular to each other (transverse and longitudinal)
- Any pathologic (or suspected pathologic) structure should have imaging attempted in at least two planes (transverse and longitudinal)

ULTRASOUND TECHNIQUE

- A full discussion of techniques to optimize image quality is beyond the scope of this textbook
- Not all ultrasound machines have the same names for components used to maximize images. Become familiar with controls and settings provided by your machine.
- Select proper ultrasound probe or probe setting using megahertz setting appropriate for level of imaging
  ○ Higher frequency ultrasound probes for superficial imaging
  ○ Lower frequency ultrasound probes for deeper imaging
- Adjust depth of imaging to localized area of interest to center of ultrasound screen – "maximize screen real estate"
- Adjust near and far gain (depth gain) setting to equalize image brightness and maximize edge delineation
- Decrease power settings to lowest available setting at which details are easily seen
- Adjust focus to correspond to area of greatest interest on the ultrasound screen
- Probes with similar megahertz settings but different crystal arrangement provide different imaging capabilities
- Tissue harmonic imaging (THI) is a setting that toggles on and off and may improve imaging capabilities
- For many machines, using color Doppler imaging will decrease temporal resolution (making the frame rate look choppy)

IMAGE DOCUMENTATION: STILL IMAGES VS. VIDEO IMAGES

Still Images (Pro)

- Framing of image occurs before image archiving (i.e., first you find the "perfect image"; then hit record)
- Easier to identify intended images during quality assurance image review (i.e., only intended images are archived)
- No external equipment is required to review still images
- Less expensive to record ultrasounds as paper or electronic stills
- Less cumbersome to set up still image quality assurance process
- False-negative ultrasounds with adequate images but inappropriate interpretation are detected during the quality assurance (QA) process
    Example: A false-negative FAST read initially as negative that shows free fluid can be re-read as a true positive during QA

Video Images (Pro)

- Easier for quality reviewer to identify errors in imaging technique of ultrasonographer
- Easier to document multiple images during ultrasound
- Image archival more representative, better documentation of entire ultrasound
- Less likely to miss documentation of pathology
  - Single-image representation of an ultrasound can miss pathologic findings
- False-negative ultrasounds due to inappropriate interpretation are detected during QA process
- Videotape review allows a tighter QA process which better identifies poor technique and gaps in knowledge and also provides an opportunity for education during tape review
- Easier to accurately interpret ultrasound despite atypical or unusual views
- Less complicated recording process results in fewer unrecorded ultrasounds in a busy emergency department
- Recording when study begins and ends allows QA review to perform "indirect observation" of scanning performance and technique in real time. This can allow greater detail in feedback to the physician learning ultrasound as the QA review can note where difficulties were occurring (e.g., scanning duodenum for 5 minutes before identifying the gallbladder).

    Although still image recording of ultrasounds may be less expensive and easier to initiate as a QA process, the positives of videotaping all ultrasounds may outweigh the negatives. Clinicians who perform bedside ultrasound will tend to perform fewer and more varied ultrasounds than dedicated ultrasound sonographers in the radiology, cardiology, gynecology, or other specialty suites. This is the nature of emergency ultrasound, and highlights why a tighter videotape QA process may better identify individuals who require further training in the performance as well as interpretation of clinical bedside ultrasound. Still image QA may be appropriate in situations where clinicians are more experienced, perform a greater number of ultrasounds, videotape review is not technically feasible, or where only a few clinicians perform ultrasound.

Basic Mechanics of Acquiring Ultrasound Images

2

Romolo Gaspari

There are four basic movements of the ultrasound probe that allow proper imaging. Every ultrasound probe has an indicator that provides a basic orientation. The orientation of the probe is indicated by a mark on the ultrasound screen. The four basic movements of the ultrasound probe are

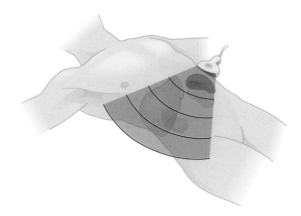

- Movement in-line with the ultrasound probe indicator—think of "sliding along" the image
- Movement perpendicular to the ultrasound probe indicator—think of "fanning through" the image
- Rotation of the probe—think of "spinning through" the image
- Movement along the axis of the probe (i.e., increased pressure on the patient's skin)—think of "pushing toward" the image
- Rocking movement without moving the probe (i.e., "heel-toeing movement")

Each of these movements causes entirely different results on the images being acquired. To make it more complicated, the orientation of the probe affects the results of moving the probe.

ULTRASOUNDING AN EGG: PROBE MOVEMENTS IN THE ABSTRACT

Throughout this chapter, there will be examples of ultrasound probe movements and how they interact with the abstract shape of an ordinary egg. By using the shape of an egg, you will better understand how moving the probe affects the images you view on the screen.

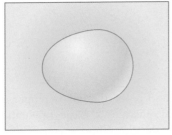

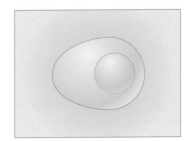

Outside of Egg   Inside of Egg

Initial Orientation

It is critical to understand where you are starting from. The ultrasound probe emits sound in a very narrow flat plane like a fan. A probe located at the epigastrium can be moved toward the umbilicus with quite different results depending on which way the indicator is located. With the indicator oriented toward the patient's head, the plane of imaging is the long axis of the body. This same location on the body with the indicator toward the patient's right side produces a plane of imaging that is the short axis of the patient's body.

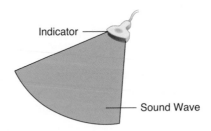

Indicator

Sound Wave

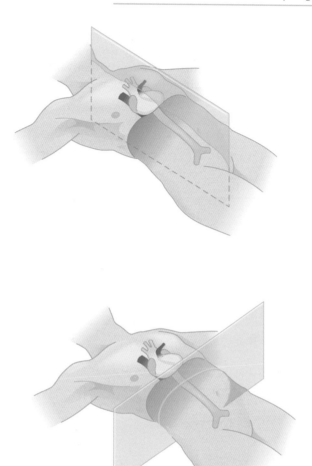

Orientation of the Egg

The egg has two true axes, unlike the human body which has three. The two axes are longitudinal and transverse. Any axis that is not long or transverse is oblique. The third axis of the human body is coronal, which in the egg is the same as longitudinal, just turned on its side.

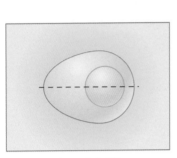

Long Axis 2D

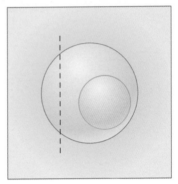

Short Axis

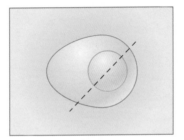

Oblique Axis

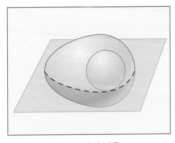

Long Axis 3D

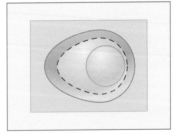

Coronal Axis

These views are obtained by orienting the probe with the indicator toward the "tip" of the egg or the "side" of the egg. Imagine cutting a hard-boiled egg along its longest axis and pulling the two halves apart to look at the yolk. This is what you are doing with the ultrasound beam when you are viewing it in the long axis. When cutting the egg in the long axis, you may have a slice with yolk in it or you may not.

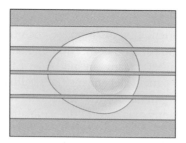

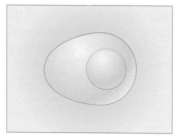

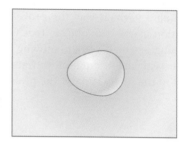

Slice # 2

Slice #4

The short axis is just like cutting the egg into round segments and seeing if you have any yolk in the segment. In the diagram below, the first three slices of egg have no yolk in them but the next three slices have yolk in their center.

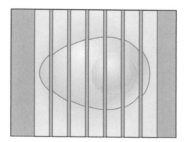

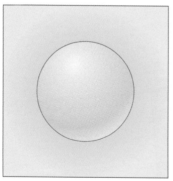

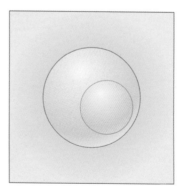

Slice #2

Slice #5

A Comment on Orientation

When commenting on the orientation of an image, the orientation refers to the object of interest, not necessarily the patient's body. Although some organs are oriented with the axis of the body (i.e., aorta), many are not (i.e., cardiac). Some organs have a variable orientation and are patient dependent (i.e., gallbladder). Therefore you may have a long axis view of the gallbladder that is actually oblique to the patient's body. This is still described as the long axis view of the gallbladder.

Sliding Along the Image

Movements of the probe toward the patient's feet will have two different effects depending on which way the probe is oriented. Moving along the axis of the probe orientation causes the objects that you are viewing to "slide" across the screen. The same thing is true if you are moving the probe from the patient's right side to patient's left side, with the orientation in transverse. The important fact is that you are moving parallel to the orientation of the probe.

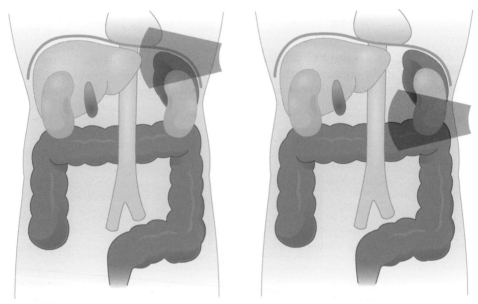

Probe Movements

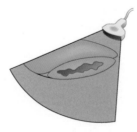

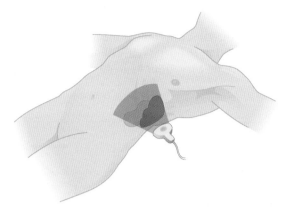

Probe Movements

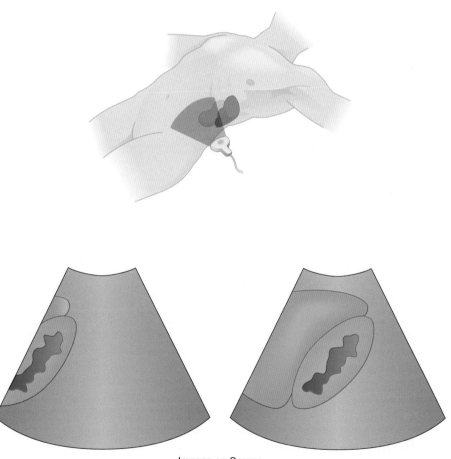

Images on Screen

Sliding Along the Egg

If the indicator is pointing the same direction as the probe is moving, the objects on the screen will remain unchanged in character but will move across the screen. Sliding the probe to the right will move the view from #1 to #2.

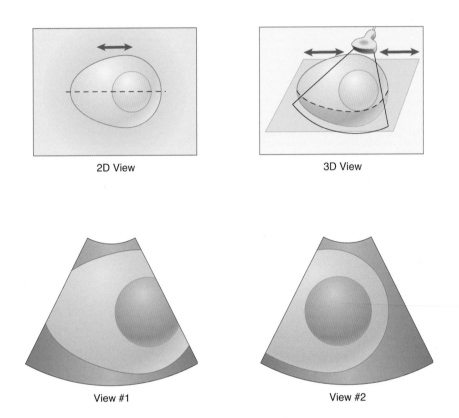

2D View   3D View

View #1   View #2

Fanning Through an Image

Doing the same movements with the probe (i.e., sliding toward the patient's feet) but changing the probe orientation to the patient's right causes different results. This movement will cause a "fanning through" of the objects on the screen. By moving the probe perpendicular to the orientation of the probe you are moving the ultrasound waves through the patient's body like a tennis racquet through the air. In the following example, you are viewing the ultrasound wave end on (like the edge of the tennis racquet). Moving the probe down the patient's side with the orientation in transverse causes the kidney to "shrink" as you scan from the thicker middle to the thinner end of the kidney.

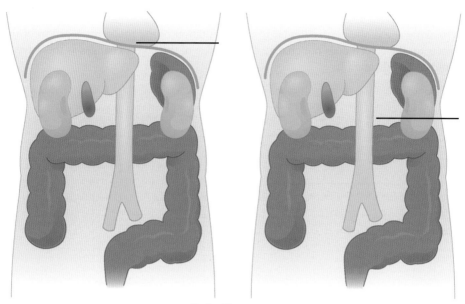

Probe Movements

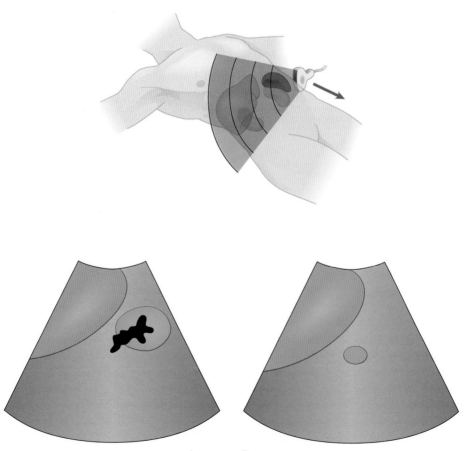

Images on Screen

Fanning Through the Egg

By moving the probe perpendicular to the orientation of the probe the location of the objects on the screen does not change, but the size of the object changes as the wave of sound passes through it.

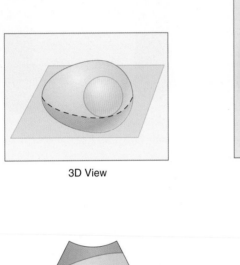

3D View

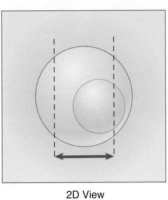

2D View

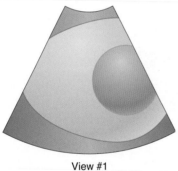

View #1

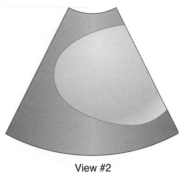

View #2

Rocking the Probe

You may also "fan through" a patient or "slide along" without actually moving the probe on the skin surface. Rocking the probe back and forth without moving the contact point with the patient's skin accomplishes the same effect as moving the entire probe up and down. Rocking in-line with the probe orientation will cause the images to slide back and forth, while rocking perpendicular to the orientation causes "fanning through."

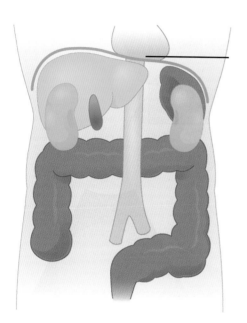

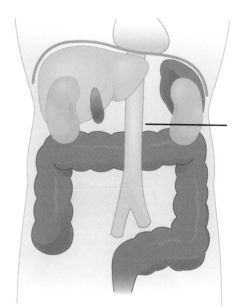

or

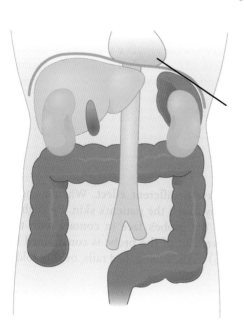

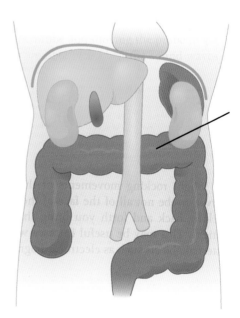

Rotating the Probe

Without moving the probe on the patient's skin but rotating it 90 degrees will cause a shift in orientation. This can be thought of as "spinning through" the image.

Note: Turning the probe 180 degrees will simply invert the image on the screen.

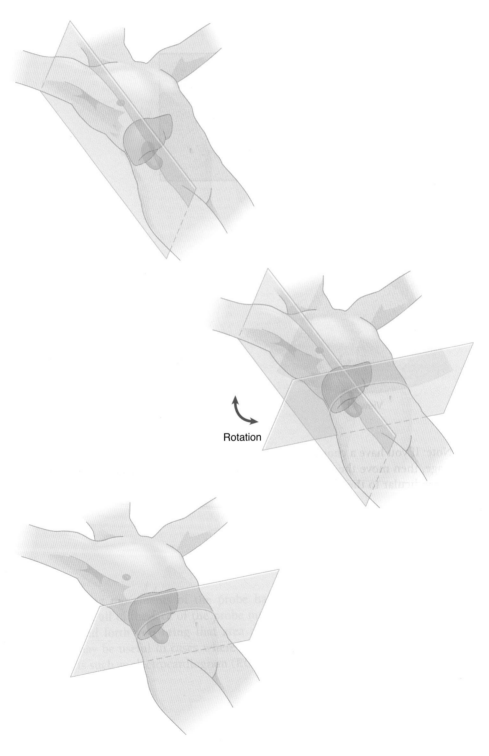

Rotation

Probe Movements

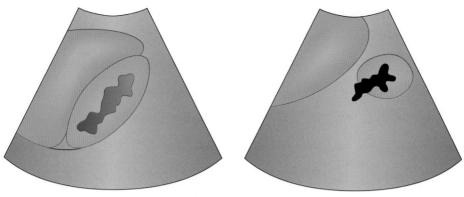

Images on Screen

As an example, think of the aorta in a longitudinal plane with the indicator toward the patient's head then rotate the indicator counterclockwise until it points to the patient's right side. The aorta is now in a transverse plane.

Note: All points in between longitudinal and transverse are termed "oblique" and are formed any time the probe is rotated to an axis that is not longitudinal or transverse (*to the item of interest, not necessarily the patient's body*).

Rotating Through the Egg

When the probe remains stationary on the surface of the egg but is rotated 90 degrees, the image on the screen will change from longitudinal or long axis to transverse or short axis.

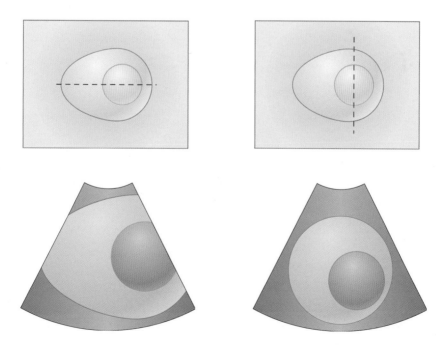

Pushing In on the Probe

By increasing pressure of the probe on the patient's skin you will move the probe toward the objects on the screen. The closer you are to an object the better the image quality will be, but increased pressure may be uncomfortable to the patient. It is very useful to get closer to the object of interest and displace something that was between the probe and the object of interest (typically the bowel). However, it is not always possible to displace the objects between the probe and what you are looking at.

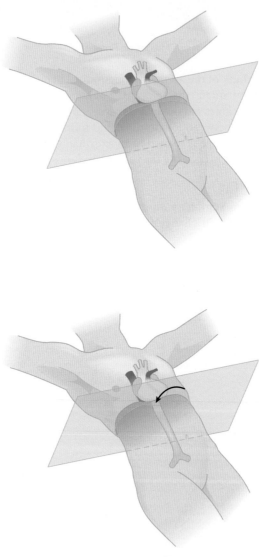

Probe Movements

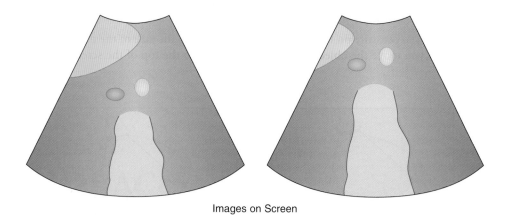

Images on Screen

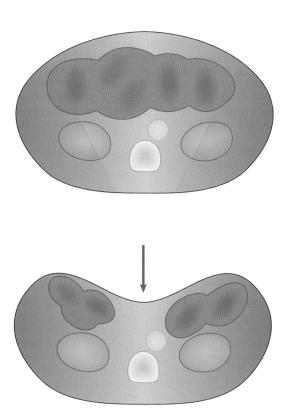

THORACO-
ABDOMINAL
PROTOCOLS

Focused Assessment Sonography of Trauma (FAST) Scanning Protocol

Romolo Gaspari

GOAL OF THE FAST EXAM

Demonstrate free fluid in abdomen, pleural space, or pericardial space.

EMERGENCY ULTRASOUND APPROACH

The focused assessment of sonography in trauma is unique for ultrasounds performed in the emergency department as it is designed as a screening assessment for patients involved in penetrating or blunt trauma. Although it is possible to use ultrasound to determine solid organ injury, the FAST scan is designed as a *screening* tool for peritoneal blood and should be used as such. Once the initial screening has been accomplished, it is possible to return to areas of interest and more fully evaluate for solid organ injury, but this should not impede patient care. Other imaging modalities are better suited to determining solid organ injury (i.e., CAT scan).

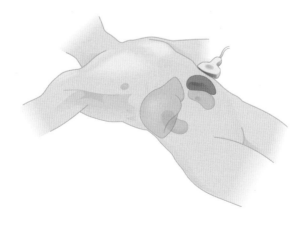

ANATOMY

The anatomy of interest in the FAST scan covers three areas of the abdomen and one of the thorax.

Right Upper Quadrant

Liver
Kidney
Diaphragm
Morison's pouch (potential space between liver and kidney)

Left Upper Quadrant

Spleen
Kidney
Diaphragm
Splenorenal recess (potential space between spleen and kidney)

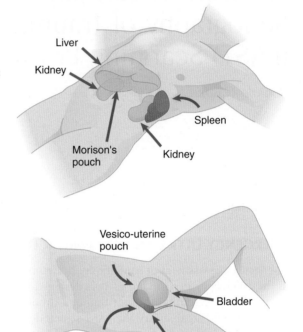

Suprapubic

Bladder
Uterus
Vesicouterine space or anterior cul-de-sac (potential space between bladder and uterus)
Rectouterine space or posterior cul-de-sac (pouch of Douglas) (potential space between uterus and rectum)

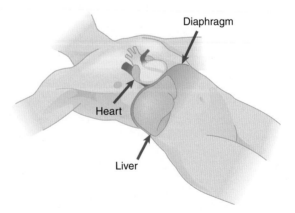

Subxiphoid/Parasternal

Liver
Diaphragm
Heart
Pericardial space (potential space around heart)

The anatomy of the abdomen during the FAST exam is unique in that the area of interest is the interface between the various abdominal or chest organs. The organs of three views of the FAST scan are used to identify the potential peritoneal spaces, but the first view identifies the pericardial space.

PATIENT POSITION

Supine

As a majority of patients are scanned following trauma, these patients will be "boarded and collared" with cervical spine and long board immobilization. There may be limited opportunity to reposition the patient secondary to concerns for cervical spine injury. In other words, the patient will be flat on his or her back and cannot be moved.

TRANSDUCER

3.0 to 5.0 MHz

Tricks of the Trade

- Deep breathing – Moves liver or spleen inferiorly and flattens the diaphragm, bringing the cardiac window closer to the subxiphoid region.

- Trendelenburg – Increases likelihood of detecting small amounts of fluid by bringing the fluid away from the air-filled bowel and into a space that is easier to view sonographically (i.e., splenorenal and hepatorenal windows).

- Infuse fluid in bladder catheter – Displaces bowel and creates a sonographic window to check for free fluid lateral and posterior to the bladder.

ULTRASOUND IMAGES

FAST Essential Images

- Subxiphoid
- Right upper quadrant (RUQ)
- Left upper quadrant (LUQ)
- Suprapubic
  (sagittal and transverse)

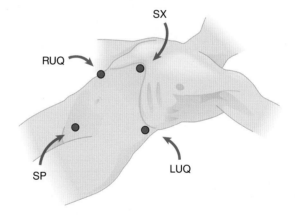

FAST Optional Images

- Right costophrenic angle
- Left costophrenic angle
- Parasternal long view of heart

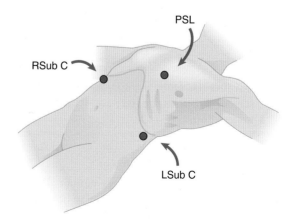

FAST: SUBXIPHOID (LONG AXIS OR SHORT AXIS)

Landmarks

- Liver–cardiac interface
- Cardiac motion

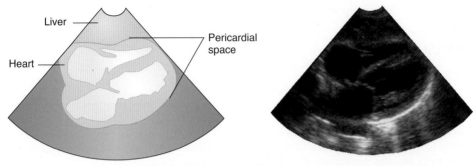

Long Axis (of Heart)

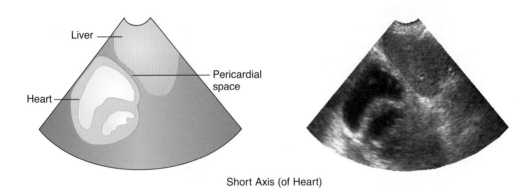

Short Axis (of Heart)

Image Elements

- Liver–cardiac interface

Tricks of the Trade

- A distended stomach following an endotracheal intubation will prevent an adequate view of the pericardium. Repeating the subxiphoid view following the placement of a nasogastric tube may improve image quality.

- Have the patient take a deep breath and hold it if possible. This will flatten the diaphragm, bring the heart closer to the probe, and improve the image.

- Advance the probe laterally along liver margin until the heart appears on the screen. This uses the liver as a window to improve visualization of the pericardium.

Partial View Probe Positioning

Note: Many of the partial views contain information that is needed to accurately identify pathology. The ideal view may be unobtainable due to patient characteristics and multiple "partial views" will be required to complete the scan.

Too Close to Xiphoid Process

Liver dominates view
Incomplete view of heart

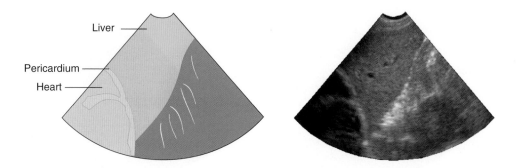

Too Far from Xiphoid Process

Liver dominates view
No or incomplete view of heart

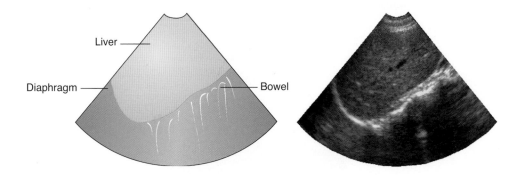

Too Far Right

Liver–pulmonary interface
No heart in view

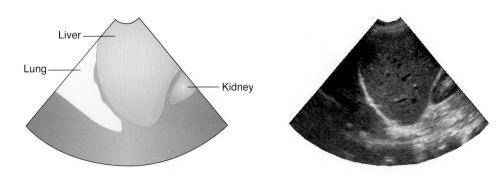

Too Far Left

No liver in image
No heart in view
Stomach gas obscures view

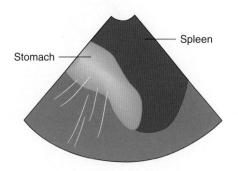 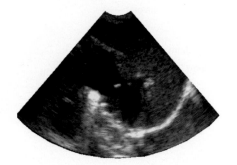

FAST: RIGHT UPPER QUADRANT

Landmarks

- Liver–kidney interface

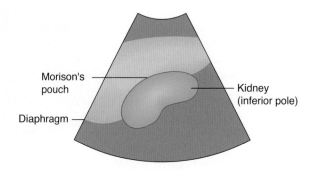

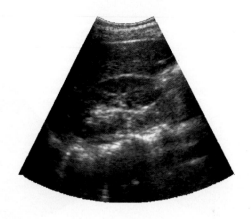

Image Elements

- Liver–kidney interface
- Diaphragm
- Inferior pole of kidney

Tricks of the Trade

- On most patients it will be necessary to slide the probe toward the head to obtain more diaphragm, and toward the feet to get down to the lower pole.

- Rib shadows represent missing information that prevents you from obtaining all the necessary information on one static image. Rather, think of it as a dynamic process that involves "seeing around" the ribs to obtain all the necessary information.

- With practice, your mind will eventually "subtract out" the rib shadows as you manipulate the probe and as the patient breathes in and out.

- Retroperitoneal blood may be visualized "deep" to the kidney.

- When performing a FAST exam do not be distracted by pathology in other organs unrelated to the traumatic event (e.g., mild hydronephrosis in the kidney).

Partial View Probe Positioning

Note: Many of the partial views contain information that is needed to accurately identify pathology. The ideal view may be unobtainable due to patient characteristics and multiple "partial views" will be required to complete the scan.

Too Cephalad

Liver dominates view
Incomplete view of Morison's pouch
Missing inferior tip of kidney, *or*
Missing inferior tip of liver, *or*
Excessive view of lung

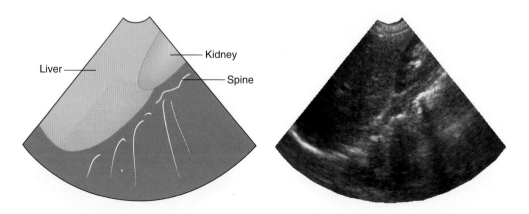

Too Caudad

Kidney on left of screen
Incomplete view of Morison's pouch
No view of diaphragm, *or*
Loops of bowel dominate image

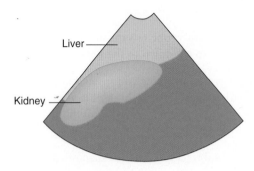 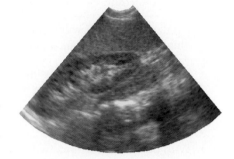

Too Medial

Liver–bowel interface dominates screen
No view of Morison's pouch
No view of kidney
(+/–) Vena cava or aorta in view

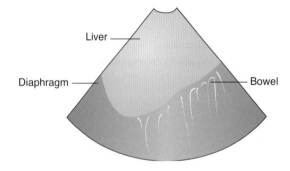 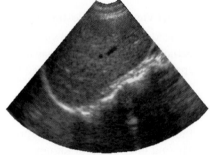

Too Lateral or Too Posterior

Kidney dominates image
Limited view of Morison's pouch
No view of diaphragm

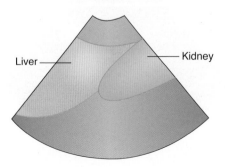 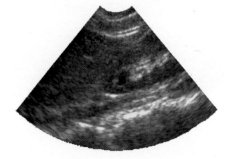

FAST: LEFT UPPER QUADRANT

Landmarks

- Liver–spleen interface

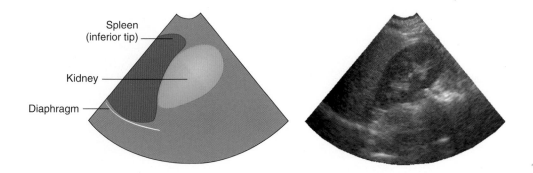

Image Elements

- Liver–spleen interface
- Diaphragm
- Inferior pole of kidney
- Inferior tip of spleen

Tricks of the Trade

- Poor images usually result from approaching the LUQ from too far anterior. In the emergency department we rarely have the luxury of a fasting patient during a trauma. A full stomach will obscure much of the kidney–spleen interface.

- Most kidneys are more posterior and superior than one might think. If you do not see the kidney, move more posterior and superior.

- Be careful of calling free fluid around the stomach. The food, fluid, gas interface in the stomach from recent eating may simulate free fluid. This will not extend to the inferior spleen which is the most common area of a positive FAST scan in the LUQ view.

- An intercostal view of the spleen–kidney interface will usually have some rib shadows. Rotating the probe 5 to 10 degrees clockwise may remove the shadow and improve your view.

- Perirenal fat may appear as a hypoechoic area between the kidney and spleen but will contain some internal echoes.

Partial View Probe Positioning

Note: Many of the partial views contain information that is needed to accurately identify pathology. The ideal view may be unobtainable due to patient characteristics and multiple "partial views" will be required to complete the scan.

Too Cephalad

Pulmonary air obscures part of view
Excessive view of lung
Spleen on right of screen

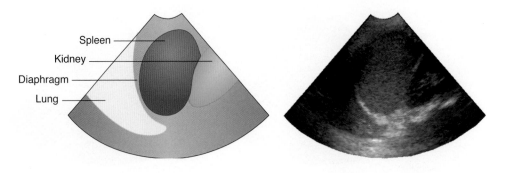

Too Caudad

Kidney on left or center of screen
No diaphragm in view

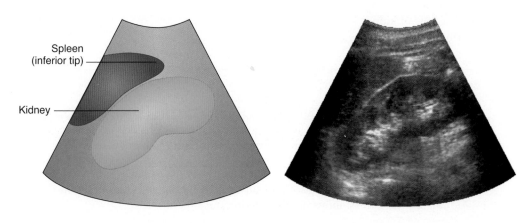

Too Medial (Anterior)

Stomach obscures view
Kidney not in view

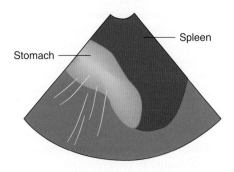 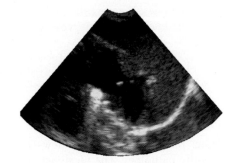

Too Posterior

Kidney dominates image
Limited view of spleen–kidney interface
No view of inferior tip of spleen

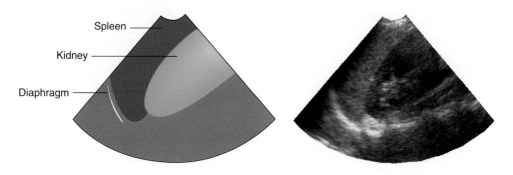

Too Shallow

Kidney dominates image
No inferior tip of spleen
No view of diaphragm

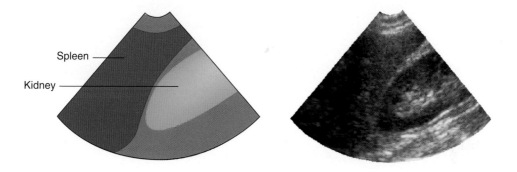

SUPRAPUBIC

Landmarks

- Bladder–uterine interface
- Bladder–bowel interface

Male Bladder Long Axis

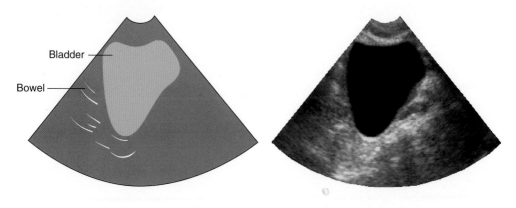

Male Bladder Transverse Axis

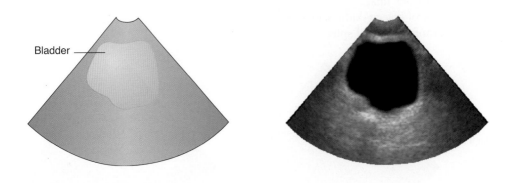

Female Bladder Long Axis

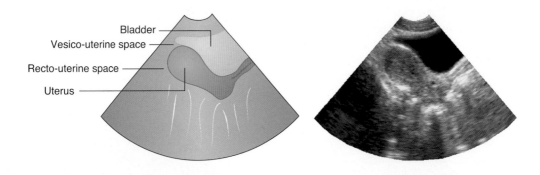

Female Bladder Short Axis

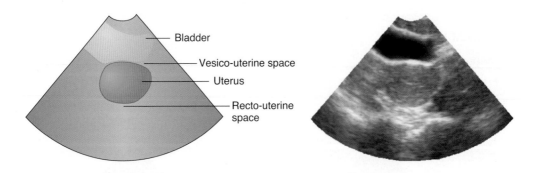

Image Elements
- Outline of bladder
- Uterine silhouette (female)

Tricks of the Trade

- Performing the suprapubic ultrasound following a bladder catheterization is extremely difficult. Either perform prior to bladder catheterization or refill bladder with saline.

- Reverse Trendelenburg will collect the available fluid in the pelvis and increase the likelihood that it will be identified. (Note: This is rarely needed.)

- Through transmission of sound through the bladder may result in the area behind the bladder being "over gained" or being too white, which can result in false negatives. This should be corrected by adjusting the time gain compensation (TGC).

- Fluid-filled bowel loops can appear as dark shapes in the pelvis but should not demonstrate the sharp angles seen with free fluid. This is easier to determine in the short axis view by imaging the bowel loops superior to the bladder.

- Blood clots within the lumen of the bladder may appear as mobile echogenic shapes or debris.

Partial View Probe Positioning

Note: Many of the partial views contain information that is needed to accurately identify pathology. The ideal view may be unobtainable due to patient characteristics and multiple "partial views" will be required to complete the scan.

Too Cephalad or Angle Too Steep

No bladder in image, *or*
Bladder on right of screen
Bowel dominates view

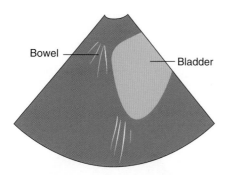
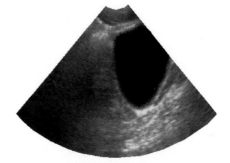

Angle Too Shallow

Pubic symphysis obscures view
Nonvisualization of internal structures

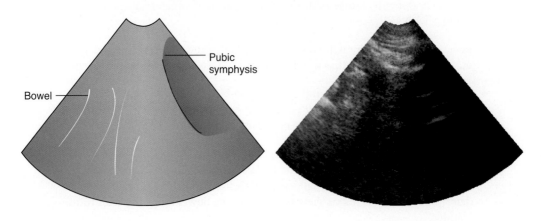

Too Caudad

Pubic symphysis partially obscures view
Bladder on left of screen

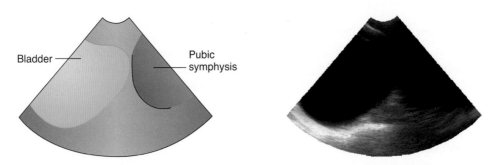

Too Far Right or Left

Bladder off-center (transverse)
Small view of bladder (long)
Bowel dominates view

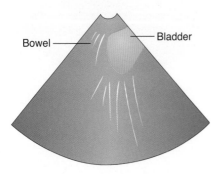
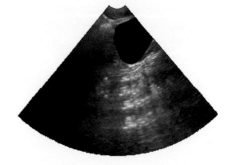

Alternative or Unusual Views

Costophrenic angle (right)
Similar to RUQ too high

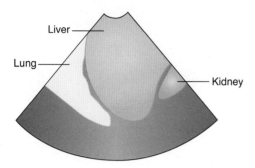 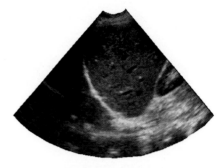

Costophrenic angle (left)
Similar to LUQ too high

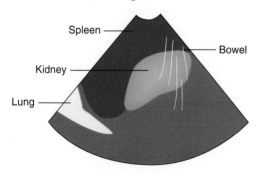 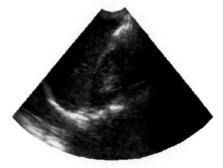

Suprapubic during catheter insertion

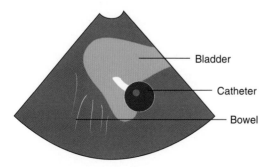 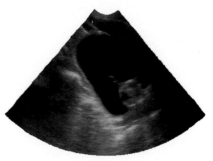

Parasternal long view of pericardium

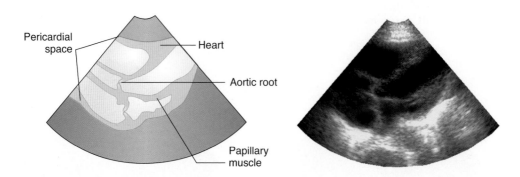

ULTRASOUND PROTOCOL TECHNIQUE

Still Image Protocol

RUQ – Sagittal plane, anterior
   Transducer at costal margin
      or lower intercostal spaces
   Right anterior axillary line
   Indicator toward patient's head
   Angle probe slightly medial

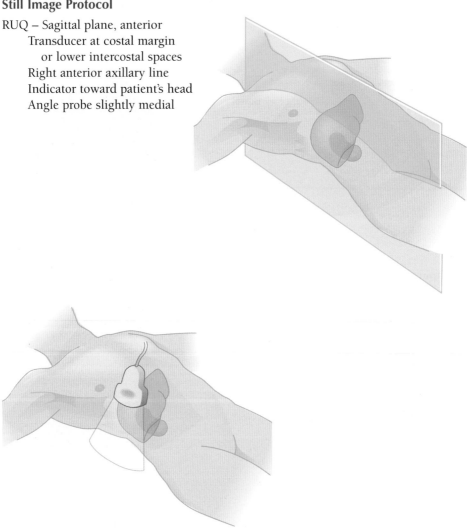

RUQ – Coronal plane, lateral
    Transducer at costal margin or lower intercostal
    Right middle axillary line
    Indicator toward patient's head
    Angle probe slightly posterior

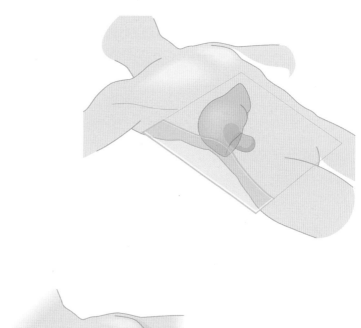

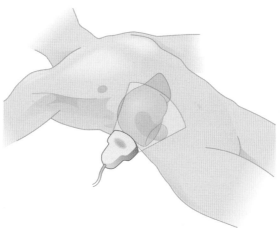

Subxiphoid – Transverse plane, anterior
  Transducer at costal margin
  Midline abdomen, subxiphoid
  Indicator toward patient's right side
  Angle probe toward right scapula

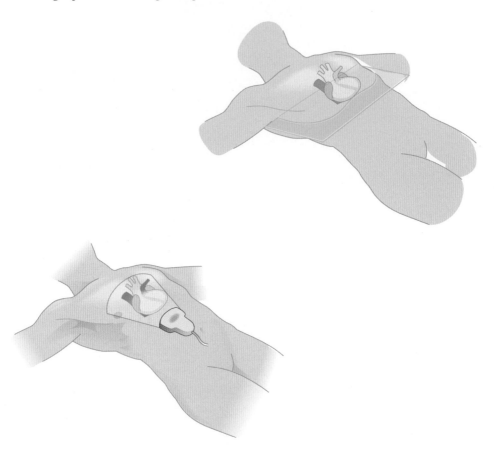

LUQ – Coronal plane, lateral
  Transducer at left intercostal
  Left posterior axillary line
  Indicator toward patient's head
  Angle probe anterior

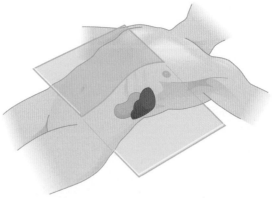

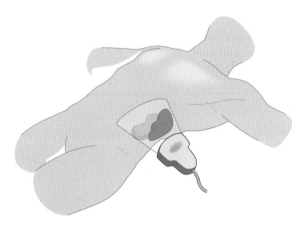

Suprapubic – Sagittal plane, anterior
   Transducer at midline abdomen
   Superior to pubic symphysis
   Indicator toward patient's head
   Angle probe inferior

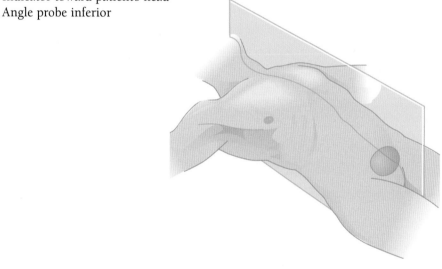

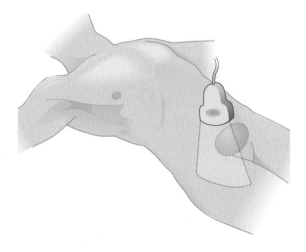

–Alternative–
Suprapubic – Transverse plane, anterior
    Transducer at midline abdomen
    Superior to pubic symphysis
    Indicator toward patient's right
    Angle probe inferior

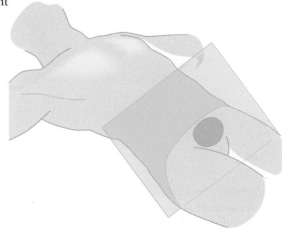

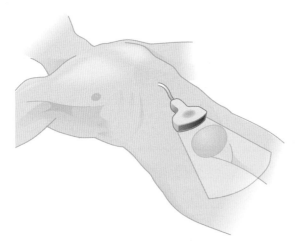

Optional Still Images

Parasternal long view of pericardial space
    Oblique plane, anterior
    Transducer at intercostal space
    Lateral to sternum, left side
    Indicator toward patient's right
        shoulder
    Probe perpendicular to
        chest wall

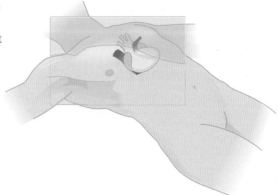

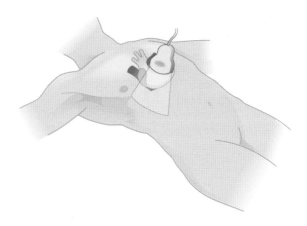

Costophrenic angle, right
    Coronal plane, lateral
    Transducer at costal margin
    Right middle axillary line
    Indicator toward patient's head
    Angle probe toward patient's head

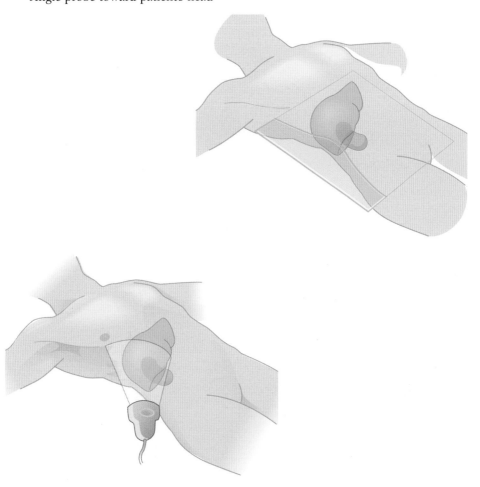

Costophrenic angle, left
    Coronal plane, lateral
    Transducer at costal margin
    Left middle axillary line
    Indicator toward patient's head
    Angle probe toward patient's head

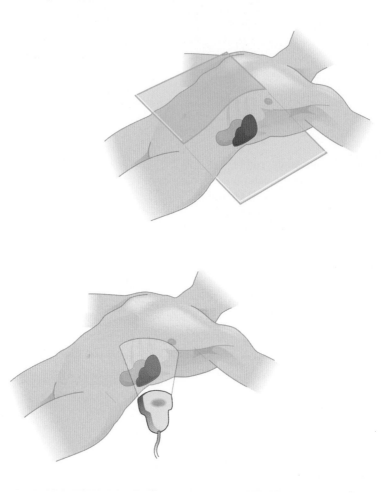

ULTRASOUND PROTOCOL TECHNIQUE

Videotape Protocol

RUQ – Starting point, sagittal plane, anterior
 Transducer at costal margin or lower intercostal
 Right anterior axillary line
 Indicator toward patient's head
 Angle probe slightly medial
RUQ – Taping protocol
 Focus on renal–liver interface
 Sweep medial to lateral
 Include view of diaphragm
 Include view of inferior kidney

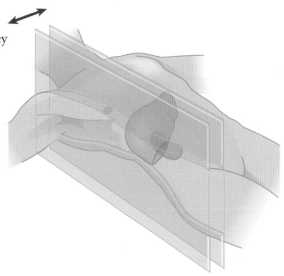

–Alternative–
RUQ – Starting point; coronal plane, lateral
 Transducer at costal margin or lower intercostal
 Right middle axillary line
 Indicator toward patient's head
 Angle probe slightly posterior
RUQ – Taping protocol
 Focus on renal–liver interface
 Sweep probe anterior to posterior
 Include view of diaphragm
 Include view of inferior kidney

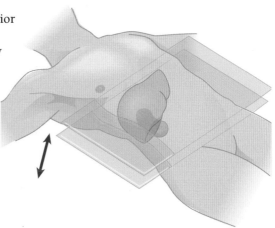

Subxiphoid – Starting point, transverse plane, anterior
    Transducer at costal margin
    Midline abdomen, subxiphoid
    Indicator toward patient's right side
    Angle probe toward right scapula
Subxiphoid – Taping protocol
    Focus on heart–liver interface
    Sweep anterior to posterior

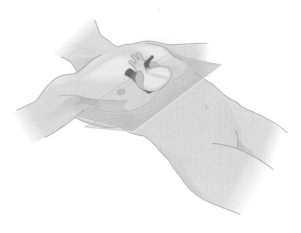

LUQ – Starting point, coronal plane, lateral
    Transducer at left intercostal
    Left posterior axillary line
    Indicator toward patient's head
    Angle probe anterior
LUQ – Taping protocol
    Focus on kidney–spleen interface
    Sweep probe anterior to posterior
    Include view of diaphragm
    Include view of inferior kidney
    Include view of inferior tip of spleen

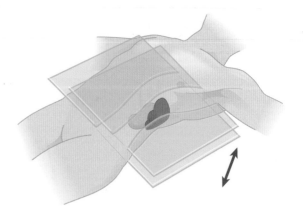

Suprapubic – Starting point, sagittal plane, anterior
> Transducer at midline abdomen
> Superior to pubic symphysis
> Indicator toward patient's head
> Angle probe inferior

Suprapubic – Taping protocol
> Focus on outline of bladder
> Sweep probe side to side
> Demonstrate retrovesicular
>> space
> Demonstrate retrouterine
>> space

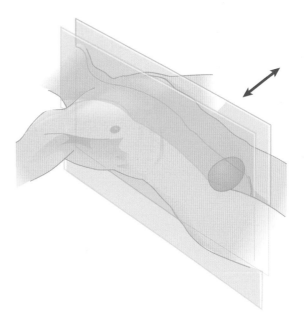

–Alternative–
Suprapubic – Starting point, transverse plane, anterior
> Transducer at midline abdomen
> Superior to pubic symphysis
> Indicator toward patient's right
> Angle probe inferior

Suprapubic – Taping protocol
> Focus on outline of bladder
> Sweep probe superior to inferior
> Demonstrate retrovesicular space
> Demonstrate retrouterine space

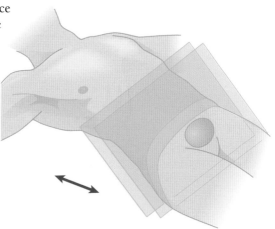

Optional Video Images

Pericardial space – Starting point, parasternal long view
 Oblique plane, anterior
 Transducer at 5th intercostal space
 Lateral to sternum, left side
 Indicator toward patient's right shoulder
 Probe perpendicular to chest wall
Pericardial space – Parasternal long tape protocol
 Focus on outer silhouette of heart
 Slight sweep from left shoulder to right hip
 Only limited movement of probe is needed

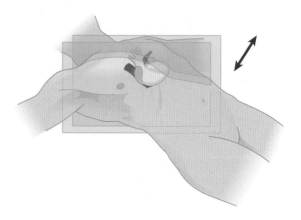

Costophrenic angle right, starting point
 Coronal plane, lateral
 Transducer at costal margin
 Right middle axillary line
 Indicator toward patient's head
 Angle probe toward patient's head
Costophrenic angle right – Tape protocol
 Focus on pleural space superior to diaphragm
 Sweep probe anterior to posterior
 Similar protocol to RUQ except
  orientation is superior

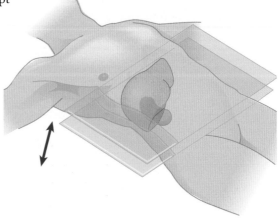

Costophrenic angle left
    Coronal plane, lateral
    Transducer at costal margin
    Left posterior axillary line
    Indicator toward patient's head
    Angle probe toward patient's head
Costophrenic angle left – Tape protocol
    Focus on pleural space superior to diaphragm
    Sweep probe anterior to posterior
    Similar protocol to LUQ except orientation is superior

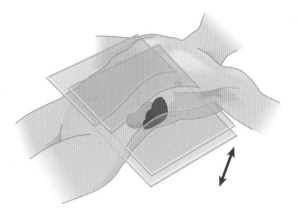

Gallbladder Scanning Protocol

Romolo Gaspari

GOAL OF GALLBLADDER ULTRASOUND

Demonstrate abnormalities in gallbladder and extrahepatic bile ducts including wall thickening, gallstones, ductal dilatations, and surrounding tissue.

Emergency Ultrasound Approach

Emergency medicine ultrasound of the gallbladder is focused on the clinical questions involving the gallbladder and common bile duct. Patients with right upper quadrant (RUQ) pain are commonly seen in the emergency department. The most common yes–no question that is addressed with an emergency medicine ultrasound of the gallbladder is whether or not there are gallstones. It is important to understand that the presence or absence of gallstones (or any other ultrasonic finding of the gallbladder) is not by itself diagnostic for biliary colic. Other questions such as evaluation of a palpable mass or the possibility of common bile duct dilation may also arise.

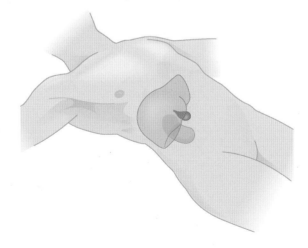

Anatomy

The anatomy of interest in the gallbladder scan involves the gallbladder and extrahepatic ductal system. The orientation of the gallbladder is variable as it is not completely tethered within the abdominal cavity. The anatomy of the extrahepatic ductal system has a number of common variations which are discussed below.

Gallbladder
    Gallbladder interior
        Body
        Fundus
        Neck
    Wall of gallbladder
Extrahepatic ductal system
    Common bile duct
    Hepatic duct
    Cystic duct
Pericholecystic space

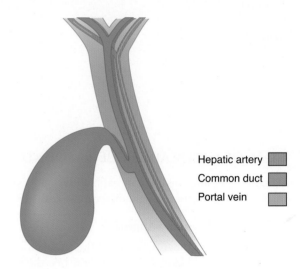

Hepatic artery
Common duct
Portal vein

(Note: For the purpose of an emergency ultrasound any portion of the extrahepatic biliary duct is referred to as the "common duct.")

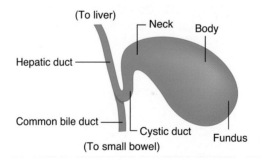

Patient Position

Supine
Sitting
Left lateral decubitus
Standing

Patient Preparation

A fasting state improves image quality.

Transducer

3.0 to 5.0 MHz.

Gallbladder Pathology

- Gallstones cause bright internal echoes with posterior shadowing that move with patient position
- Sludge causes a dependent hypoechoic (but not anechoic) layer
- Gallbladder wall thickening is defined as when the gallbladder wall measures more than 3 to 5 mm
- Fluid around the gallbladder forms an anechoic rim or band
- Gallbladder pathology, such as gallstones and sludge, is independently mobile of other gallbladder anatomy. Imaging of the gallbladder should be performed in multiple patient positions.

Common Duct Pathology

- The common duct normally measures less than 5 mm or 40% of associated portal vein but is larger in older individuals
- Internal echoes within the lumen of the common duct may represent common duct stones

Maneuvers

Deep breaths (or pushing out abdominal wall) may lower the gallbladder below the costal margin.

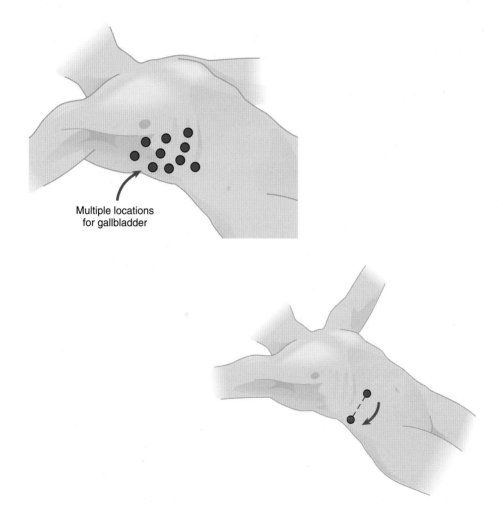

Multiple locations
for gallbladder

Locating the Gallbladder

- Multiple locations due to patient variation
- Start at epigastrium and sweep along costal margin
- Consider intercostal approach

Locating the Common Duct

- Locate portal triad in liver parenchyma
- Locate neck of gallbladder
  - Image anterior to portal vein

Tricks of the Trade

- Using a deep, wide initial sweep – Shows relative association between organs in the RUQ.

- Deep breathing – Lowers the diaphragm causing the inferior edge of the liver to drop below the costal margin, improving image quality.

- Patient positioning affects the location of the gallbladder – Sitting patient up, left lateral decubitus, standing. Changing patient position can improve image quality.

- Gallbladder wall should be measured at anterior gallbladder due to increased artifact of posterior wall.

- Gallbladder contracts following eating resulting in thickening of the gallbladder wall and decrease in gallbladder size.

ULTRASOUND IMAGES

Gallbladder Essential Images

- Gallbladder long axis
- Gallbladder short axis
  - Neck of gallbladder
  - Body of gallbladder
  - Fundus of gallbladder

Gallbladder Optional Images

- Common duct long axis
- Common duct short axis

GALLBLADDER LONG AXIS

Landmarks

- Main lobar fissure
- Portal triad

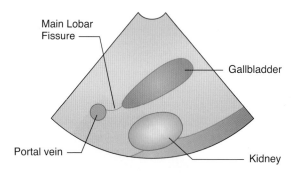

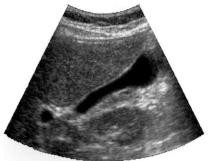

Image Elements

• Contour of gallbladder
• Internal architecture of gallbladder
• Pericholecystic space

Additional Information Obtained During Imaging

• Gallbladder wall thickness
• Common bile duct width

Tricks of the Trade

• Drinking water prior to imaging gallbladder will decrease duodenal bowel gas and improve image quality.

• Orientation of gallbladder is variable – Once it is located, oblique probe slightly back and forth to identify true long axis.

• Gas–fluid interface of duodenum mimics gallbladder with gallstones. To tell the difference, (1) watch for peristalsis, (2) image gallbladder in at least two planes, and (3) look for another "gallbladder."

Partial View Probe Positioning

Note: Many of the partial views contain information that is needed to accurately identify pathology. The ideal view may be unobtainable due to patient characteristics and multiple "partial views" will be required to complete the scan.

Too Cephalad

Liver dominates view
Gallbladder on right of screen
Gallbladder fundus not seen

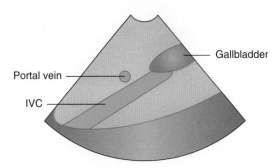

Gallbladder

Portal vein

IVC

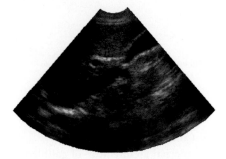

Too Caudal

Limited liver tissue in view (no landmarks)
Gallbladder on left of screen
(+/–) Small bowel dominates screen
Poor image quality

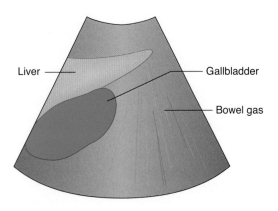

Liver

Gallbladder

Bowel gas

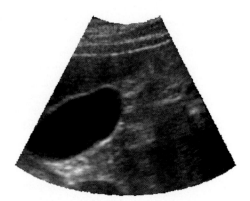

Too Medial

Liver dominates view
No gallbladder in view

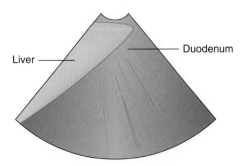

Liver

Duodenum

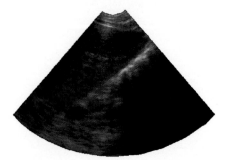

Too Lateral

Liver–renal interface dominates view
No gallbladder in view

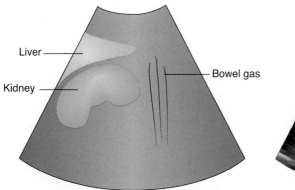
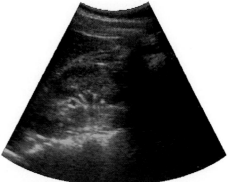

Too Deep

Gallbladder small and at top of image

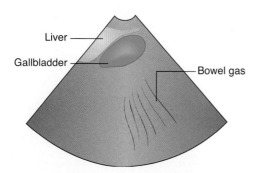
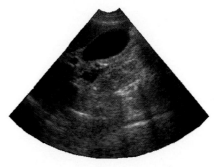

GALLBLADDER SHORT AXIS (NECK, BODY, AND FUNDUS VIEWS)

Landmarks

- Superior pole of kidney

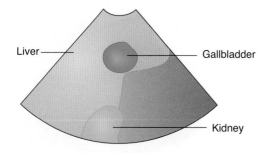
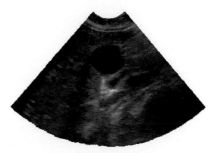

(Note: Superior pole of kidney is not always in same view as gallbladder.)

Image Elements

- Gallbladder contour
- Gallbladder wall
- Internal gallbladder architecture
- Pericholecystic space

Tricks of the Trade

- Clearly demonstrate landmarks in at least one view of transverse gallbladder. Some landmarks are not readily visualized in all transverse images of the gallbladder.

- The transverse gallbladder is essentially an anechoic circle. Other anechoic circles seen in the RUQ can confuse the novice sonographer (portal vein, inferior vena cava, fluid-filled duodenum, etc.). Rotating the probe 90 degrees will differentiate the gallbladder from other vascular structures.

Neck of Gallbladder

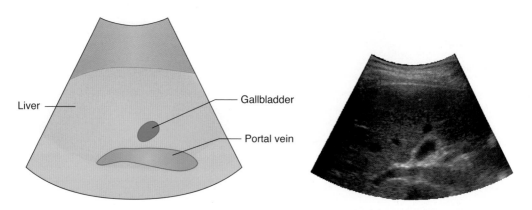

Body of Gallbladder

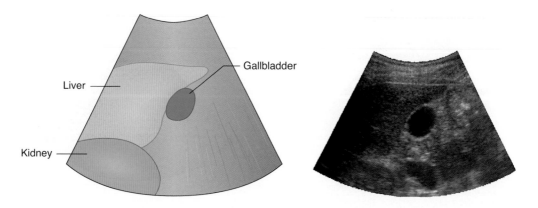

Fundus of Gallbladder

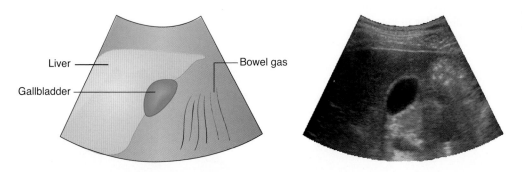

Partial View Probe Positioning

Note: Many of the partial views contain information that is needed to accurately identify pathology. The ideal view may be unobtainable due to patient characteristics and multiple "partial views" will be required to complete the scan.

Too Cephalad

Liver dominates image
No gallbladder in view

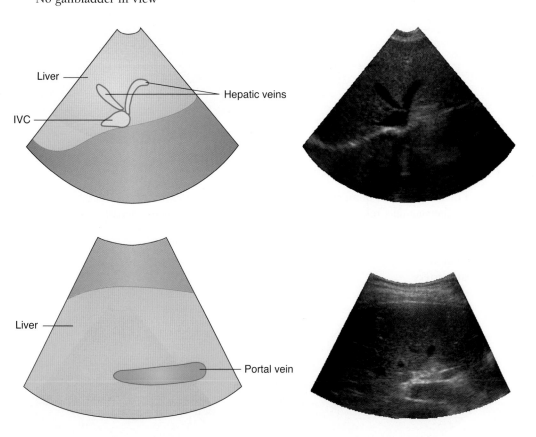

Too Caudad

Bowel loops dominate image
No gallbladder in view
Poor image quality

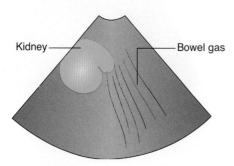
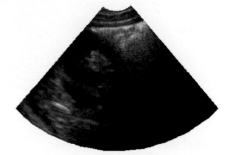

Too Medial

Liver dominates view
Vena cava or aorta in view (+/−)
Gallbladder on left of screen (+/−)

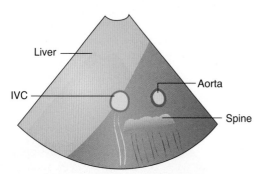
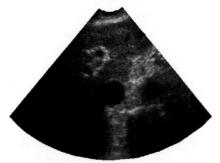

COMMON DUCT LONG AXIS

Note: For the purposes of an emergency ultrasound of the extrahepatic ductal system, the term *common duct* refers to either the common bile duct or the hepatic duct.

Landmarks

- Portal vein
- Hepatic artery

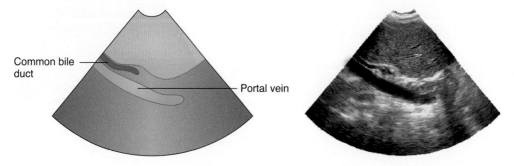

Distal Common Duct

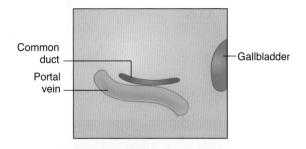

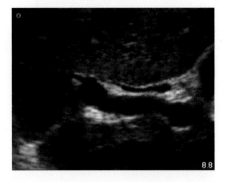

Proximal Common Duct

Image Elements

- Portal triad
  - Portal vein
  - Common duct
  - Hepatic artery
- Images of common duct vary by location along course of common duct
  - Distal common duct
    - Portal vein and common duct run parallel to each other
  - Proximal common duct
    - Hepatic artery may course in between a parallel common duct and portal vein

---

Tricks of the Trade

- Imaging portal vein and common duct through liver parenchyma allows for higher image quality.

- Identify the portal triad at the neck of the gallbladder in transverse orientation, rotate to long axis, and trace distally.

- Doppler can distinguish hepatic artery from common duct.

Partial View Probe Positioning

All poor probe positioning will cause loss of visualization of common duct with either liver or small bowel dominating view.

COMMON DUCT SHORT AXIS

Landmarks

- Portal triad
- Neck of gallbladder
- Main lobar fissure

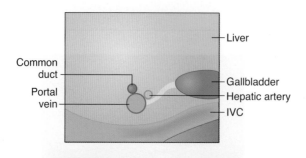

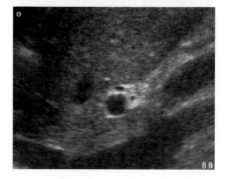

Image Elements

- Portal triad
  - Portal vein
  - Common duct
  - Hepatic artery

    Relationship of the components of the portal triad vary by location along course of portal vein.

Tricks of the Trade
• Locating the portal triad is more difficult than performing the actual protocol.
• Lateral cystic shadowing may cause artifact that crosses the portal triad at the neck of the gallbladder.
• Additional information can be obtained by imaging the distal common duct. After locating the common duct, trace it distally toward small bowel.

Partial View Probe Positioning

- All improper probe positioning will cause loss of visualization of common duct
- Liver or small bowel dominates view

Finding the Common Duct

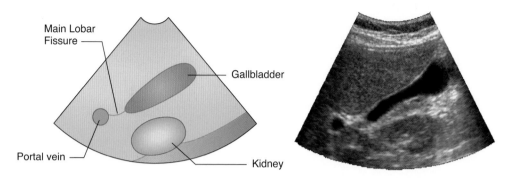

Using a long axis view of the gallbladder allows identification of the main lobar fissure which leads to the portal vein. Center probe on portal triad. Optimizing image quality and image layout will increase visualization of the common duct.

ULTRASOUND TECHNIQUE

Still Image Protocol
Gallbladder: Long Axis

Approach – Sagittal or oblique plane, anterior
Variable – Transducer at costal margin or intercostal
Variable – Anterior midclavicular line
Indicator toward patient's head or right shoulder
Probe perpendicular to skin

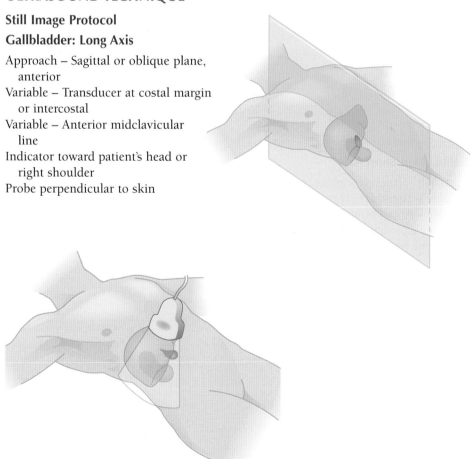

–Alternative–

Approach – Coronal plane, lateral

Variable – Transducer at lower intercostals

    Midaxillary line

    Indicator toward patient's head

    Probe perpendicular to skin

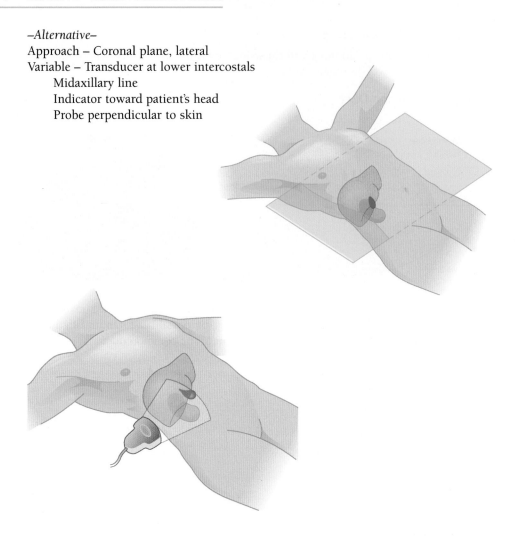

Gallbladder: Short Axis

Approach – Transverse plane, anterior

Variable – Transducer at costal margin or intercostal

Variable – Anterior midclavicular line

    Indicator toward patient's right side

    Probe perpendicular to skin

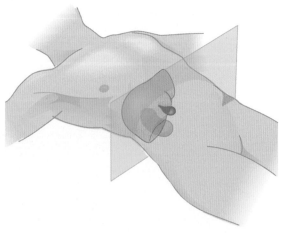

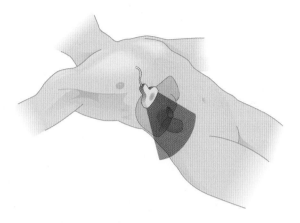

Common Bile Duct or Hepatic Duct: Long Axis

Approach – Oblique plane, anterior
    Transducer at left intercostals or subcostal
    Anterior midclavicular line
    Indicator toward patient's head or right shoulder
    Probe perpendicular to skin

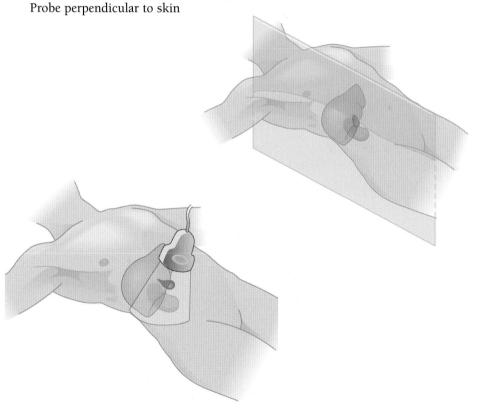

Common Bile Duct or Hepatic Duct: Short Axis

Approach – Oblique plane, anterior
     Transducer at left intercostals or subcostal
     Anterior midclavicular line
     Indicator toward patient's head or left shoulder
     Probe perpendicular to skin

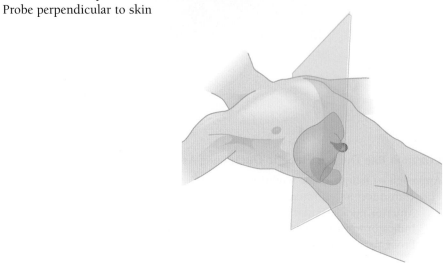

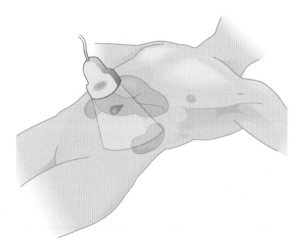

VIDEOTAPE PROTOCOL

Gallbladder: Long Axis

Starting point – Oblique plane, anterior
    Transducer at left intercostals or subcostal
    Anterior midclavicular line
    Indicator toward patient's head or right shoulder
    Probe perpendicular to skin

Taping protocol
    Focus on longest axis of gallbladder
    Sweep medial to lateral and back
    Include entire length of gallbladder
    Sweep entire width of gallbladder

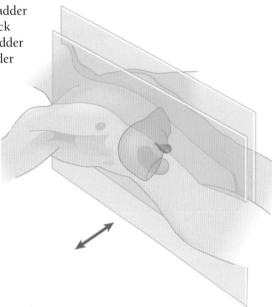

–Alternative–
Starting point – Coronal plane, lateral
    Transducer at lower intercostals or costal margin
    Middle axillary line
    Indicator toward patient's head
    Probe perpendicular to skin

Taping protocol
    Focus on longest axis of gallbladder
    Sweep anterior to posterior and back
    Include entire length of gallbladder
    Sweep entire width of gallbladder

Gallbladder: Short Axis

Starting point – Transverse plane, anterior
Variable – Transducer at costal margin or intercostal
Variable – Anterior midclavicular line
    Indicator toward patient's right side
    Probe perpendicular to skin

Taping protocol
    Focus on gallbladder
    Sweep superior to inferior
    Include entire width of gallbladder
    Sweep entire length of gallbladder

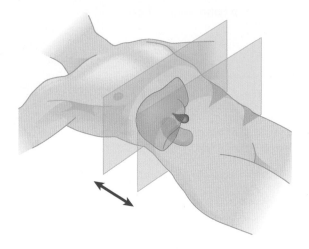

Common Bile Duct or Hepatic Duct: Long Axis

Starting point – Oblique plane, anterior
    Transducer at left intercostals or subcostal
    Midclavicular line
    Indicator toward patient's right shoulder
    Probe perpendicular to skin

Taping protocol
    Focus on parallel portal vein and common duct
    Measure diameter of common duct

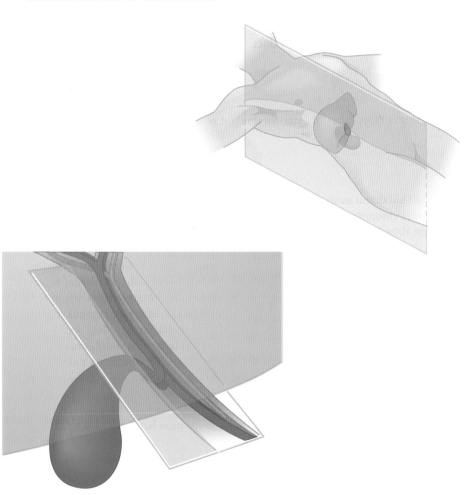

PATIENT POSITION

Supine
Left lateral decubitus
Right lateral decubitus

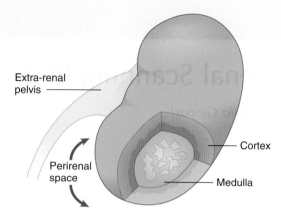

PATIENT PREPARATION

A full bladder assists in evaluation of the bladder.

TRANSDUCER

3.0 to 5.0 MHz

MANEUVERS

Inserting a catheter and filling the bladder with fluid will assist in evaluating the bladder for some patients.

RENAL PATHOLOGY

- Hydronephrosis results in interconnecting anechoic spaces in the center of the kidney
- Renal cysts result in round anechoic spaces in the parenchyma of the kidney
- Renal stones in the body of the kidney result in bright echoes with posterior shadowing.

(Note: Stones in the parenchyma of the kidney do not cause renal colic pain.)

ULTRASOUND IMAGES

Renal Essential Images

- Right kidney long axis
- Right kidney short axis
  - Superior pole
  - Middle pole
  - Inferior pole

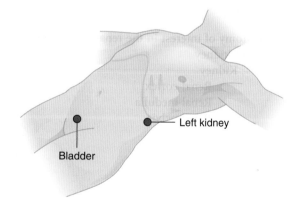

- Left kidney long axis
- Left kidney short axis
  - Superior pole
  - Middle pole
  - Inferior Pole
- Bladder
  - Long axis
  - Transverse axis

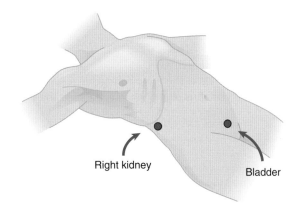

Right kidney

Bladder

Tricks of the Trade

- If only one view of the kidney is possible, the long axis view including the renal collecting system provides the most clinical information.

- When rotating the probe with the image of the kidney in the center of the ultrasound screen, the absolute longest length of the kidney is the true long axis.

RIGHT KIDNEY LONG AXIS

Landmarks

- Kidney silhouette

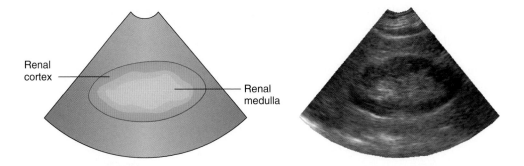

Renal cortex

Renal medulla

Image Elements

- Longitudinal view of right kidney
  - Renal pelvis
  - Renal medulla
- Perinephric space

Image Characteristics

- Kidney contour
- Kidney internal architecture
  - Cortex – medulla
  - Collecting system
- Kidney echogenicity
  - Renal pelvis is the most echogenic structure of all abdominal organs
  - Renal cortex is slightly less echogenic than the adjacent liver parenchyma

---

Tricks of the Trade

- When images are obscured by bowel gas, improvements in image quality may be seen by moving the probe posterior.

- Echogenicity of the kidney can be altered with gain adjustments. To evaluate the kidney for hypo- or hyperechogenicity, compare it to the adjacent liver.

- With true long axis of the kidney, slow rotation of the probe should shorten the length of the kidney. If it lengthens, then you know that you are slightly oblique.

- The kidney is not tethered in the abdominal cavity. As the diaphragm contracts and relaxes during normal respirations, the kidney moves up and down.

- Having the patient take a deep breath and hold it will allow improved windows for imaging the kidney.

Partial View Probe Positioning

Note: Many of the partial views contain information that is needed to accurately identify pathology. The ideal view may be unobtainable due to patient characteristics and multiple "partial views" will be required to complete the scan.

Too Cephalad

Kidney on right of screen
Incomplete view of kidney – lower pole missing

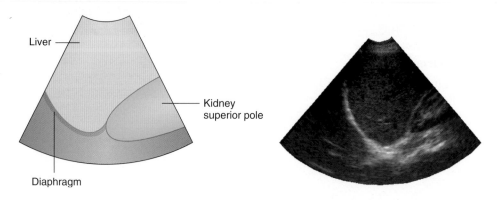

Too Caudad

Kidney on left of screen
Incomplete view of kidney – superior pole missing

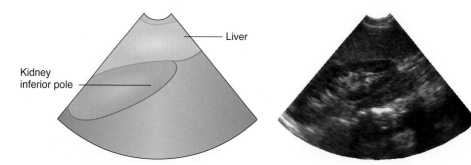

Too Medial

No kidney seen
Liver–bowel interface dominates image, *or*
Gallbladder in view, *or*
Vena cava in view, *or*
Aorta in view

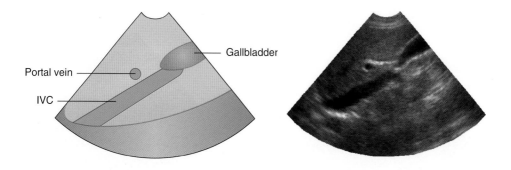

Too Anterior

Bowel loops dominate image, *or*
Kidney small and deep in image

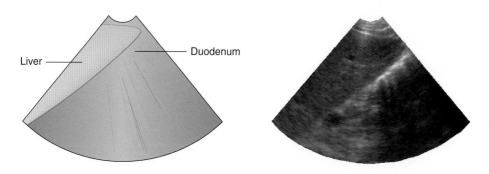

Oblique View

Kidney with bulbous, asymmetric shape.

Kidney migrates across screen with fanning through long axis.

When moving from sagittal to parasagittal, the location of the kidney should not move on the ultrasound screen.

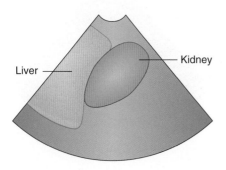
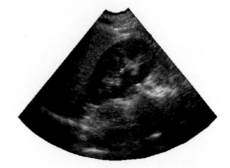

RIGHT KIDNEY SHORT AXIS

Landmarks

- Kidney silhouette
- Gallbladder (+/–)

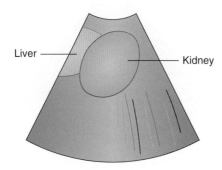
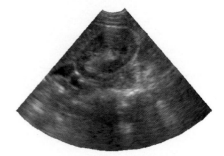

Image Elements

- Kidney contour
- Kidney internal architecture
  - ○ Cortex
  - ○ Medulla
  - ○ Collecting system
  - ○ Kidney echogenicity
- Perinephric space

Images

- Upper pole of right kidney

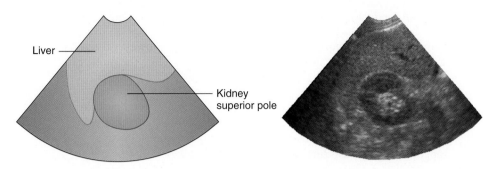

- Middle pole of right kidney

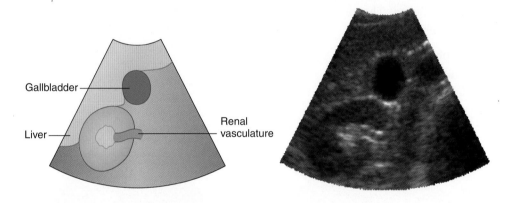

- Lower pole of right kidney

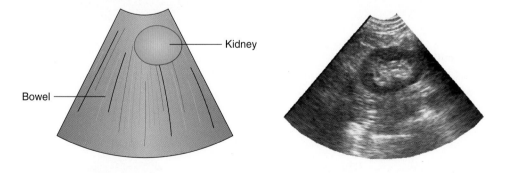

Tricks of the Trade

- If you are unsure that you have true transverse, find the true longitudinal view and rotate 90 degrees counterclockwise.

- Imaging of the superior pole when it is just under the lowest rib can be accomplished by either moving intrathoracic and angling the probe caudad, or, moving subcostal and angling the probe cephalad.

- Pathology of the kidney (tumors and cysts, etc.) may extend past the inferior or superior pole. To ensure visualization of the entire transverse kidney the kidney must *disappear* as the probe moves superior during imaging of the upper pole or inferior during imaging of the lower pole.

Partial View Probe Positioning

Note: Many of the partial views contain information that is needed to accurately identify pathology. The ideal view may be unobtainable due to patient characteristics and multiple "partial views" will be required to complete the scan.

Too Cephalad

Liver dominates image
No kidney in view

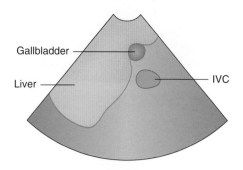
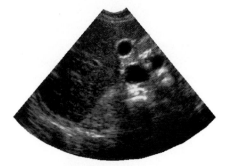

Too Caudad

Bowel loops dominate image
Poor image quality
No kidney in view

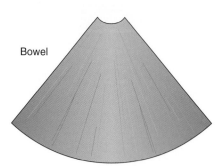
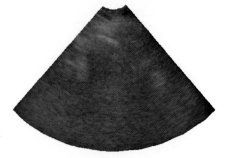

Too Medial

Kidney on left of screen, *or*
Liver–bowel interface, *or*
Vena cava in view, *or*
Aorta in view

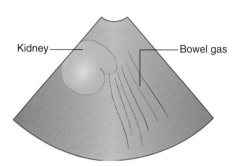
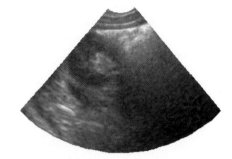

LEFT KIDNEY LONG AXIS

Landmarks

• Kidney silhouette

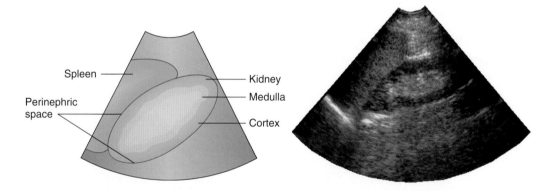

Image Elements

• Kidney contour
• Kidney internal architecture
  ◦ Cortex
  ◦ Medulla
  ◦ Collecting system
• Kidney echogenicity – Compare to splenic parenchyma
• Perinephric space

Tricks of the Trade

- The left kidney is higher and more posterior than the right.

- When rib shadows interfere with long axis imaging the left kidney, rotating the probe 5 degrees clockwise may improve imaging.

- It is not always possible to view the entire long axis of the kidney. It is sometimes necessary to image the superior and inferior poles separately in the long axis.

- Fluid in the stomach can sometimes form sharp angles due to interfacing with stomach contents and may be confused with perinephric fluid.

- Air in the stomach degrades image quality when viewing the left kidney. To improve image quality either move the probe posterior, using the spleen as a window, or have the patient drink water to displace stomach air.

Partial View Probe Positioning

Note: Many of the partial views contain information that is needed to accurately identify pathology. The ideal view may be unobtainable due to patient characteristics and multiple "partial views" will be required to complete the scan.

Too Cephalad

Kidney on right of screen
Lower pole missing

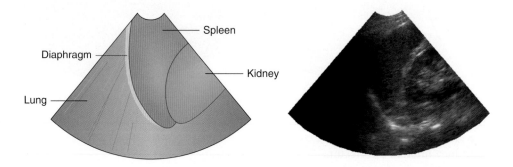

Too Caudad
Kidney on left of screen
Superior pole missing

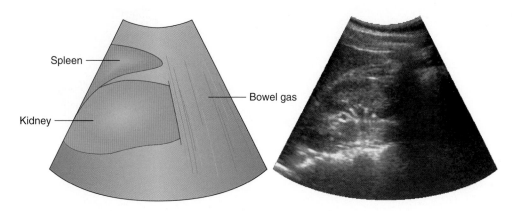

Too Medial or Anterior
Poor image quality
Stomach dominates view

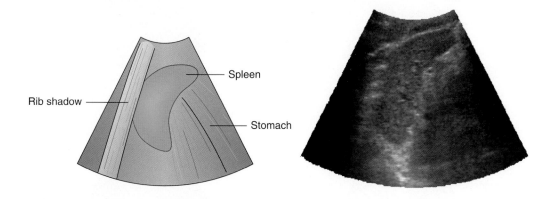

LEFT KIDNEY SHORT AXIS

Landmarks
• Kidney silhouette

Image Elements
• Kidney contour
• Kidney internal architecture
  ◦ Renal cortex
  ◦ Renal medulla
  ◦ Renal collecting system
• Kidney echogenicity
• Perinephric space

Images

• Upper pole of left kidney

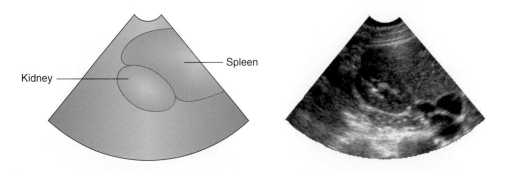

• Middle pole of left kidney

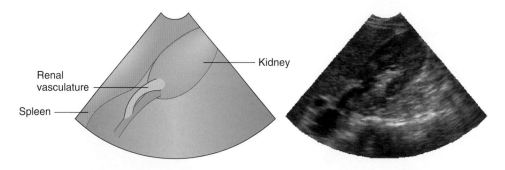

• Lower pole of left kidney

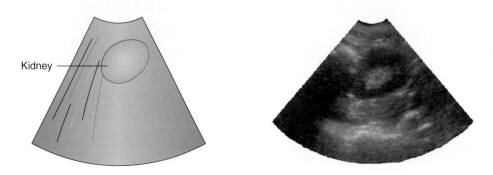

Tricks of the Trade

• Deep inspirations will lower the kidney and allow easier imaging of the superior pole.

• Right lateral decubitus positioning allows better access for imaging in patients with "thoracic" kidneys.

- A stomach with gas in it will degrade images while a stomach with fluid in it may improve images. Having the patient drink liquid may displace gas in stomach.

- Pathology of the kidney (tumors and cysts, etc.) may extend past the inferior or superior pole. To ensure visualization of the entire transverse kidney the kidney must *disappear* as the probe moves superior during imaging of the upper pole or inferior during imaging of the lower pole.

Partial View Probe Positioning

Note: Many of the partial views contain information that is needed to accurately identify pathology. The ideal view may be unobtainable due to patient characteristics and multiple "partial views" will be required to complete the scan.

Too Cephalad

Spleen dominates view, *or*
Lung dominates view, *or*
No kidney in view

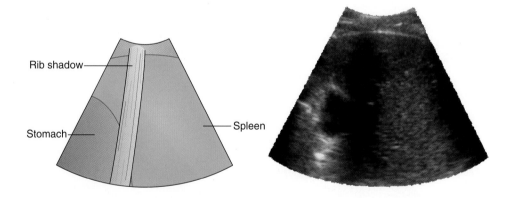

Too Caudad

Bowel loops dominate view
No kidney seen
Poor images

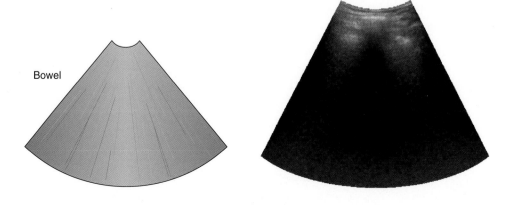

Too Medial or Too Anterior

Poor image quality
Stomach dominates view
Kidney on right of image

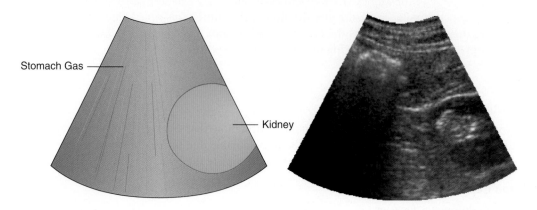

Bladder
Bladder long axis

Landmarks

- Bladder silhouette
- Bladder–uterine interface
- Bladder–bowel interface

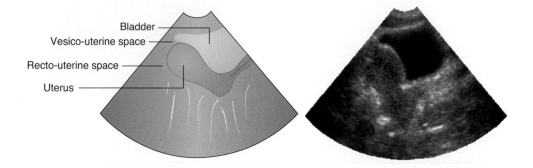

Image Elements

- Bladder contour
- Internal bladder architecture
- Retrovesicular space

Tricks of the Trade

- Anterior/posterior orientation of the uterus in female patients will change depending on degree of bladder distention.

- The most common error when the bladder is not visualized is that the probe is too superior.

- An empty bladder or one with only a small amount of urine is difficult to visualize.

Partial View Probe Positioning

Note: Many of the partial views contain information that is needed to accurately identify pathology. The ideal view may be unobtainable due to patient characteristics and multiple "partial views" will be required to complete the scan.

Too Cephalad or Angle Too Steep

No bladder in image, *or*
Bladder on right of screen, *or*
Bowel dominates view

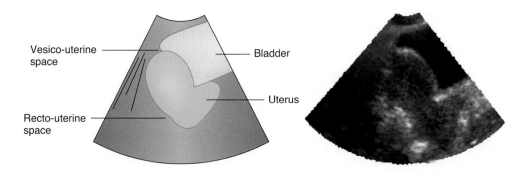

Too Caudad or Angle Too Shallow

Pubic symphysis obscures view
Poor image quality

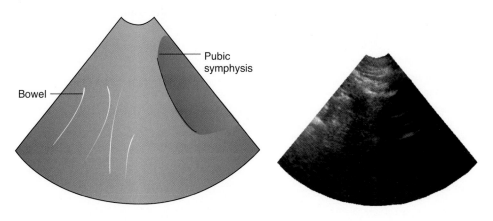

BLADDER SHORT AXIS

Landmarks

- Bladder silhouette

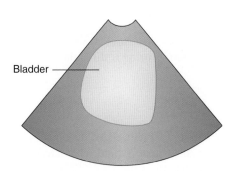 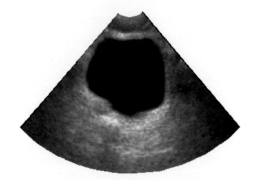

Image Elements

- Bladder silhouette
- Retrovesicular space
- Internal bladder architecture

Tricks of the Trade

- Imaging the retrovesicular space is easier with a full bladder. To fill the bladder you can have the patient drink fluids, or if there is a bladder catheter you can clamp the catheter.

- It is uncomfortable to push on a full bladder. Limit the amount of pressure when imaging the bladder transabdominally.

Partial View Probe Positioning

Note: Many of the partial views contain information that is needed to accurately identify pathology. The ideal view may be unobtainable due to patient characteristics and multiple "partial views" will be required to complete the scan.

Too Cephalad or Angle Too Steep

No bladder in image
Bowel dominates view
Poor image quality
Images will look similar if too caudad

Too Caudad or Angle Too Shallow

Pubic symphysis obscures view
No view of bladder
Poor image quality

Too Lateral or Medial

Bladder off center
Full silhouette of bladder not seen

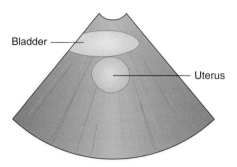
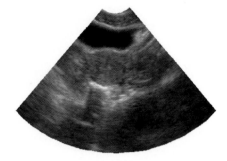

ALTERNATIVE OR UNUSUAL VIEWS

Rib Shadows

When viewing either kidney it may be partially obscured by rib shadows. Moving the probe will effectively move the rib shadow so that all of the kidney may be visualized.

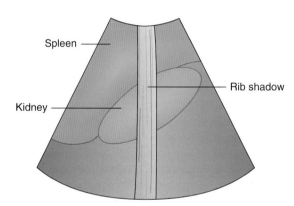
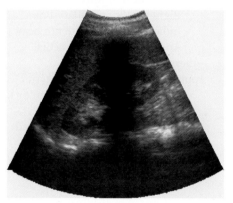

Obese Patients

Patients with a large amount of intraperitoneal fat may have perirenal fat that separates the kidney from the liver.

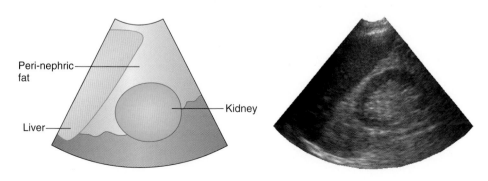

Inferior Pole Obscured

The duodenum on the left and the splenic flexure of the colon on the right may each obscure the inferior pole of the kidney.

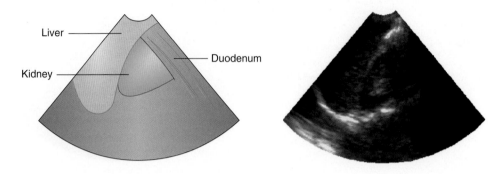

ULTRASOUND TECHNIQUE

Still Image Protocol

Right Kidney: Long Axis

Approach – Sagittal plane, oblique posterior
    Transducer at lower intercostals or costal margin
    Right posterior axillary line
    Indicator toward patient's head
    Angle probe slightly medial
–Alternative–
Approach – Sagittal plane, anterior
    Transducer at costal margin or lower intercostal
    Right anterior axillary line
    Indicator toward patient's head
    Angle probe slightly medial

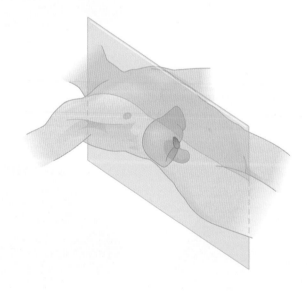

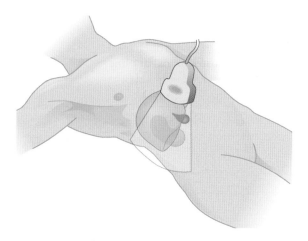

–Alternative–
Approach – Coronal plane, lateral
    Transducer at costal margin or lower intercostal
    Right middle axillary line
    Indicator toward patient's head
    Angle probe slightly posterior

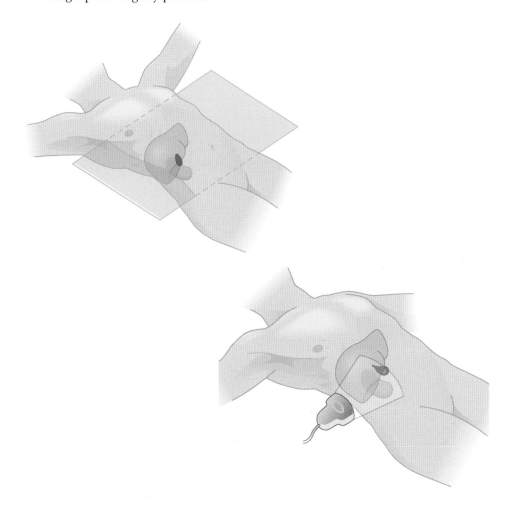

Right Kidney: Short Axis

Approach – Transverse plane, right lateral
   Transducer at costal margin or lower intercostal
   Right anterior, middle, or posterior axillary line
   Indicator toward patient's back or right side
   Probe perpendicular to skin

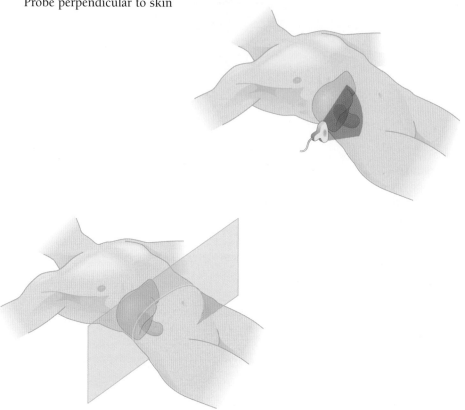

Left Kidney: Long Axis

Approach – Coronal plane, lateral
   Transducer at left intercostal
   Left posterior axillary line
   Indicator toward patient's head
   Angle probe anterior

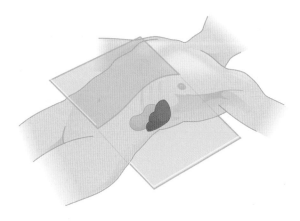

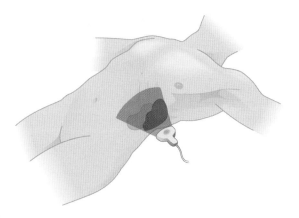

Left Kidney: Short Axis

Approach – Transverse plane, left lateral
    Transducer at left intercostal or subcostal
    Left posterior axillary line
    Indicator toward patient's front
    Probe perpendicular to skin

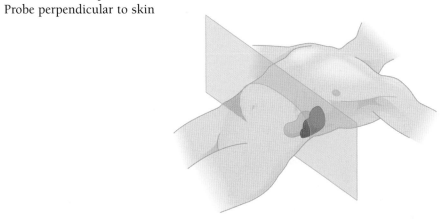

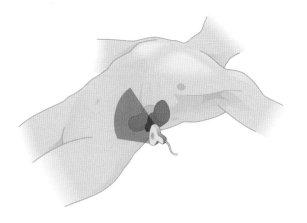

BLADDER

Bladder: Long Axis

Approach – Sagittal plane, anterior
    Transducer at midline abdomen
    Superior to pubic symphysis
    Indicator toward patient's head
    Angle probe inferior

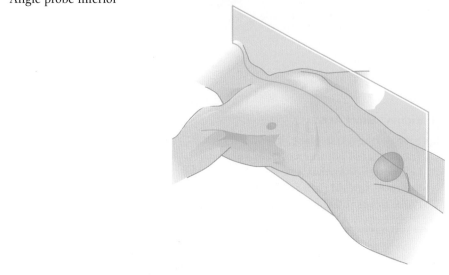

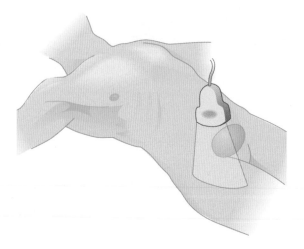

Bladder: Transverse Axis

Approach – Transverse plane, anterior
    Transducer at midline abdomen
    Superior to pubic symphysis
    Indicator toward patient's right
    Angle probe inferior

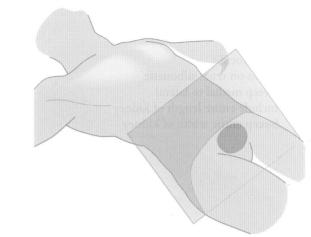

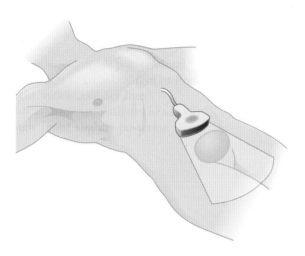

Right Kidney: Short Axis

Starting point – Transverse plane, right lateral
 Transducer at lower intercostals or costal margin
 Right posterior, middle, or anterior axillary line
 Indicator toward patient's right side or back
 Probe perpendicular to skin

Taping protocol
 Focus on renal silhouette
 Sweep superior to inferior
 Include entire width of kidney
 Sweep entire length of kidney

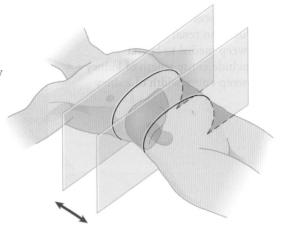

Left Kidney: Long Axis

Starting point – Coronal plane, lateral
 Transducer at left intercostal
 Left posterior axillary line
 Indicator toward patient's head
 Angle probe anterior

Taping protocol
 Focus on kidney silhouette
 Sweep probe anterior to posterior
 Include full length of kidney
 Sweep full width of kidney

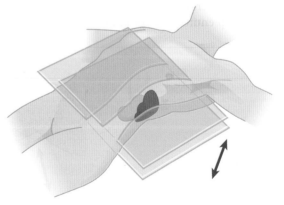

Cardia

Paul Sierzens

GOAL OF C/

Demonstrate f(
Specifically:
1. Presence of
2. Identify or (
3. Identify "im
4. Identify *glol*
5. Measure the

EMERGENCY

Emergency ca
questions invo
threatening co
yes–no questic
when patients
or heart. Patie
seen in the em

ANATOMY

The anatomy
pericardium.
1. Cardiac cha
   • Left ventr
   • Right ven
   • Left atriu
   • Right atri
2. Pericardial s
3. Cardiac valv
   • Aortic val
   • Mitral val
   • Tricuspid

Left Kidney: Short Axis

Starting point – Transverse plane, left lateral
>   Transducer at left intercostal
>   Left posterior axillary line
>   Indicator toward patient's front
>   Probe perpendicular to skin

Taping protocol
>   Focus on kidney silhouette
>   Sweep probe superior to inferior
>   Include full width of kidney
>   Sweep full length of kidney

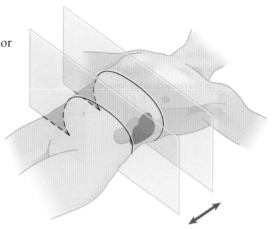

BLADDER

Bladder: Long Axis

Starting point – Sagittal plane, anterior
>   Transducer at midline abdomen
>   Superior to pubic symphysis
>   Indicator toward patient's head
>   Angle probe inferior

Taping protocol
>   Focus on outline of bladder
>   Sweep probe side to side
>   Demonstrate retrovesicular
>   space

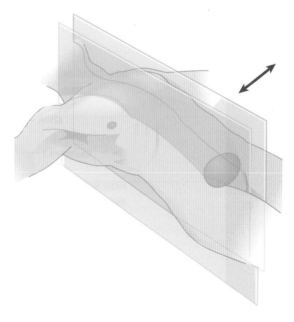

–Alternativ

Bladder: T

Starting po
    Trans
    Super
    Indica
    Angle

Suprapubi

Focus on
Sweep pro
Demonstra

PATIENT POSITION

Supine
Left lateral decubitus
Sitting

PATIENT PREPARATION

Not applicable

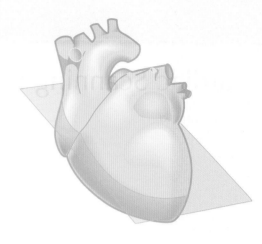

TRANSDUCER

- 2.0 to 5.0 MHz micro-convex or phased array
- A smaller transducer "footprint" or area of contact with the skin allows better visualization of the heart through the ribs

MANEUVERS

- Sitting up or left lateral decubitus will bring heart forward and improve image quality
- Deep breaths will flatten diaphragm and may improve images in subxiphoid view

CARDIAC PATHOLOGY

- Pericardial effusions result in an anechoic rim of fluid around the heart
- Wall motion abnormalities result in restricted or no movement of areas of the heart

    (Note: A full discussion of the ultrasonographic findings in patients with focal wall motion abnormalities is beyond the scope of this book.)

- Disease of the ascending aorta (i.e., aortic dissection) may result in widening of the aorta distal to the aortic valve (the aortic root)

    (Note: The cardiac ultrasound performed in the emergency department is a limited ultrasound that is designed to detect some of the emergent conditions seen in the emergency department. If any questions concerning pathology in the heart or pericardium are not adequately resolved, then a complete echocardiogram of the heart should be performed by a trained specialist.)

ULTRASOUND CARDIAC IMAGES

- Subxiphoid
- Parasternal long
- Parasternal short
- Apical two chamber
- Apical four chamber

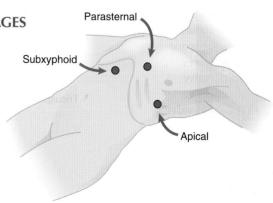

CARDIAC ESSENTIAL IMAGES

There is no set of required images for emergency medicine cardiac ultrasound, as the ultrasound may be done for a variety of reasons. For example, during a cardiac arrest, any one view of the heart that demonstrates the absence of cardiac activity is sufficient. Other applications such as the evaluation of dyspnea require additional views. In general, most emergent cardiac pathology may be identified, verified, or excluded with a 4-chamber view (either subxiphoid or apical four chamber), a parasternal long axis view, and a parasternal short axis view. Any abnormality should be verified by more than one view or window.

Tricks of the Trade

- Small pericardial effusions and pericardial fat pads present as anechoic areas adjacent to the heart. The diameter of a pericardial effusion should change during systole and diastole.

- More than one view is often required to confirm the presence of a pericardial effusion.

SUBXIPHOID

Landmarks

- Liver (when visualized)
- Cardiac silhouette
- Right ventricle (should be the most near-field chamber)

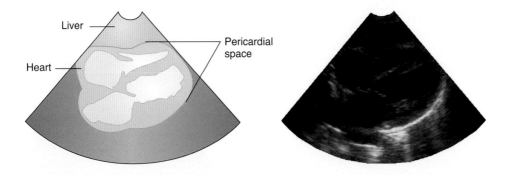

Image Elements

- Hepatic capsule/pericardial reflection
- Right ventricle

Tricks of the Trade

- Stomach contents can degrade image quality when the ultrasound probe is in the epigastrium. Moving the probe to the anterior right costal margin will improve image quality.

> • Maximize the depth setting to include the entire heart on the ultrasound screen.
>
> • It may be difficult or even impossible to get a subxiphoid view in a patient with a distended abdomen as is commonly seen following the endotracheal intubation of a patient in cardiac arrest.

Partial View Probe Positioning
Too Caudal, Too Steep of Angle, or Too Shallow Range of View

Liver dominates view
Heart at bottom of screen or not seen

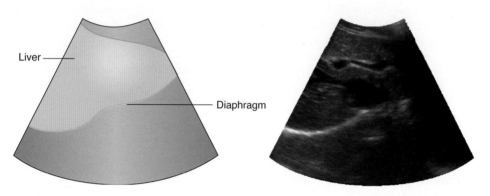

Too Lateral Right

Liver dominates view
Heart not seen

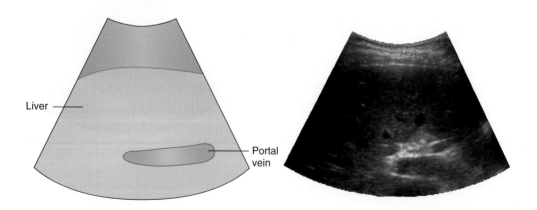

Right ventricle

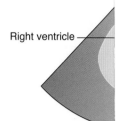

Image Elements

- Aortic valve
- Aortic root
- Left ventricle a
- Right ventricle

Tricks of the T

- The easiest
  rotate the p

Apical Four Cha

Landmarks

- Cardiac silhou
- Left ventricle
- Right ventricle

Right ventric

Tricuspid valve
Right atrium
Left atrium

Image Elements

- Left ventricle
- Right ventricle
- Left atrium
- Right atrium

Too Lateral Left

Stomach gas artifact obscures view of heart
No liver seen
Poor image quality

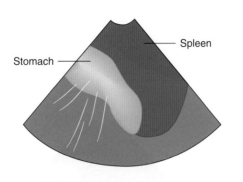

Spleen

Stomach

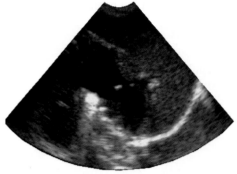

Parasternal long

Landmarks

- Cardiac silhouette
- Aortic root
- Descending thoracic aorta (DTA)

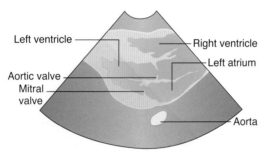

Left ventricle — Right ventricle

Left atrium

Aortic valve
Mitral valve

Aorta

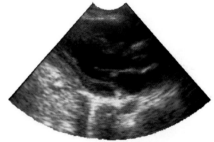

Image Elements (in One View)

- Left ventricle
- Left atrium
- Aortic valve
- Mitral valve
- Right ventricle
- Descending thoracic aorta

Tricks of the Trade

- Patients with chronic obstructive pulmonary disease (COPD) tend to have a cardiac axis that is more vertical than horizontal. They also have poor image quality due to increased air between the heart and sternum.

Parasternal S

There are thi
distal):
1. At the leve
2. At the leve
3. At the leve

Landmarks

- Cardiac sill
- Papillary n
- Aortic valv

Right ver

Tricuspid valve

Right arium

Aortic valve

Left atrium

Right ventricle

Apical Two Chamber

Landmarks

- Cardiac silhouette
- Left ventricle
- Left atrium

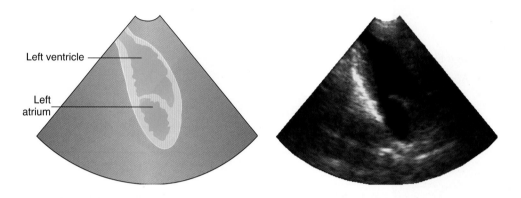

Left ventricle

Left atrium

Image Elements

- Left ventricle
- Left atrium

ULTRASOUND TECHNIQUE

Due to the inherent motion of the heart (when beating), videotape archiving of ultrasound images of the heart are easier to interpret. Much of the pathology of the heart is not apparent on still images. For example, with still images ultrasound pictures of a beating heart look identical to pictures of a heart in asystole.

It is important to understand the machine pre-sets for cardiac imaging. When obtaining cardiac images the machine can be in the 'cardiac' pre-set mode or in another mode (such as 'abdominal' pre-set). The machine automatically flips the image during 'cardiac' imaging and will indicate this by showing the direction indicator to the right of the screen. You could functionally obtain the same images in the 'abdominal' settings if you were to flip the orientation of the ultrasound probe 180 degrees. All of the orientations provided in this text assume that you are imaging with the ultrasound machine in the 'cardiac' mode.

Still Image Protocol

- If still images of the cardiac exam are to be used they should include one for each image obtained [e.g., subxiphoid/subcostal view (SUBX), parasternal long axis (PSLAX), PSSAX, etc.]
- Cardiac anatomic structures should be clearly identifiable

- A systolic and a diastolic image should be obtained, especially if a pericardial effusion or focused pathology is identified
- If a patient is in cardiac arrest, then at least three sequential, timed images should be obtained

Video Image Protocol

- If video images of the cardiac exam are to be used then each image listed below should be obtained (e.g., SUBX, PSLAX, PSSAX, etc.)
- Cardiac anatomic structures should be clearly identifiable
- All cardiac videotape protocols involve little to no actual movement of the probe once the image is perfected
- Any probe movements are for the purpose of clearing up a specific section of the ultrasound image or including an area of the heart that is not on the screen
- For each image obtained a number of sequential cardiac cycles should be included (systole and diastole)

Cardiac: Subxiphoid/Subcostal View (SUBX)

Approach – Coronal, oblique inferior
    Transducer under anterior ribs
    Epigastrium or right subcostal
    Transducer indicator toward patient's left side
    Probe angled toward left shoulder or head

Cardiac: Parasternal Long Axis (PSLAX)

Approach – Oblique plane, anterior
    Transducer left parasternal, intercostal
    Indicator toward patient's right shoulder or head
    Probe perpendicular to skin

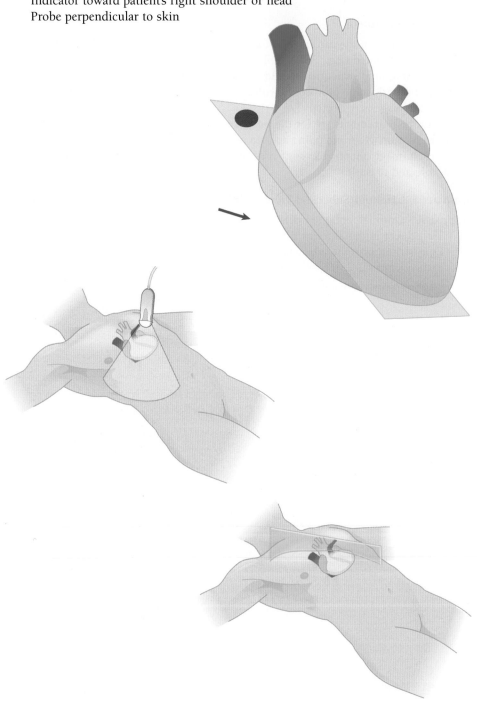

Cardiac: Parasternal Short Axis (PSSAX)

Approach – Oblique plane, anterior
 Transducer left parasternal, intercostal
 Indicator toward patient's left shoulder or left side
 90 degrees clockwise rotation from the PSLAX
 Probe perpendicular to skin
 Move probe superior–inferior
  (moves from aortic root to mid-ventricle)

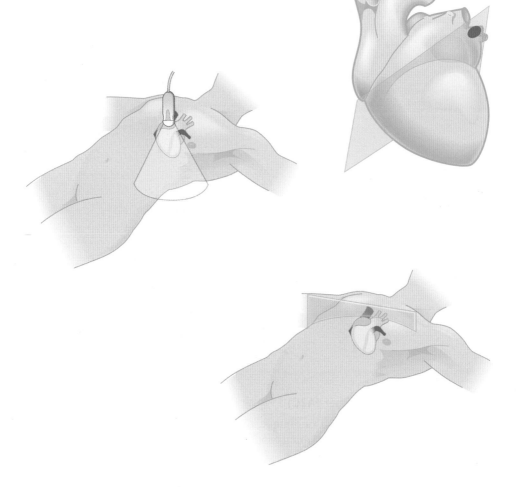

Cardiac: Apical Four Chamber (A4C)

Approach – Coronal plane, anterior oblique
  Transducer subcostal or low intercostals
  Left mid-clavicular line
  Indicator toward patient's right side
  Angle probe toward left hip
    (indicator to left axilla)

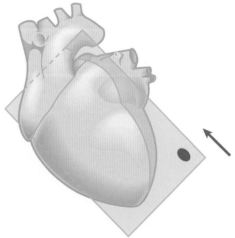

Cardiac: Apical Two Chamber (A2C)

Approach – Sagittal plane, anterior oblique
  Transducer subcostal or low intercostal
  Left mid-clavicular line
  Indicator toward ceiling
  Angle probe toward left hip
    (point toward right shoulder)

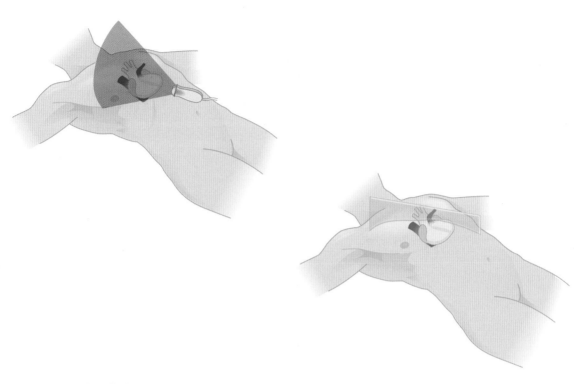

Optional Views

Suprasternal notch – Long (or short axis)
     View of aortic arch
Approach – Coronal superior (or sagittal)
     Transducer above clavicular heads
     Indicator toward head (or left side)
     Angle probe inferior

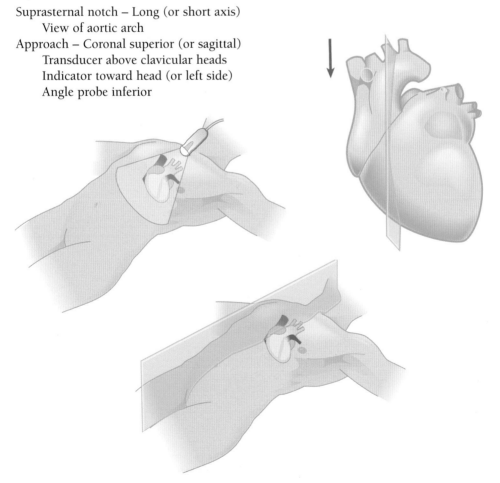

Subxiphoid short axis (note, this is a two-chamber view)
  Approach – Sagittal plane, anterior
    Transducer under anterior ribs
    Epigastrium or right subcostal
    Indicator toward patient's head or ceiling
    Probe angled toward right shoulder or head

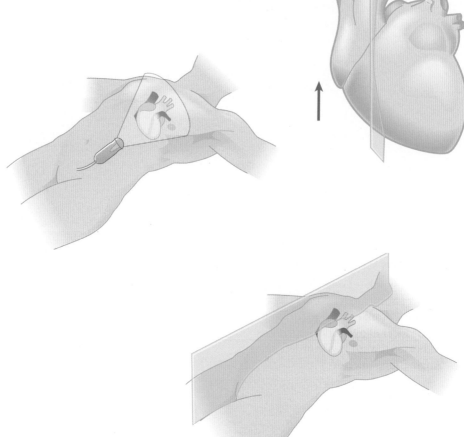

PELVIC PROTOCOLS

First Trimester Scanning Protocol

J. Christian Fox

GOAL OF A FIRST TRIMESTER ULTRASOUND

Demonstrate abnormalities in first trimester pregnancy focusing on abnormal intrauterine pregnancies or ectopic pregnancies. Recognize normal ovarian structures to differentiate these from abnormal adnexal masses.

EMERGENCY ULTRASOUND APPROACH

Emergency medicine ultrasound during the first trimester is focused on the clinical questions involving the growing embryo. Patients with bleeding during the first trimester are commonly seen in the emergency department. The most common yes–no questions addressed for these patients are those pertaining to ectopic pregnancy. The approach to imaging the uterus during the first trimester can be transabdominal or endovaginal.

ANATOMY

The anatomy of interest in the first trimester ultrasound involves the uterus. In the upright female the pelvis is tilted at 45 degrees. The uterus has a variable orientation as it is tethered at only one end. The ultrasound will focus on the contents of the uterus and the surrounding tissues.

Uterus
    Fundus
    Body
    Cervix
    Endometrial cavity
    Ovary
Bladder
Retrovesicular space

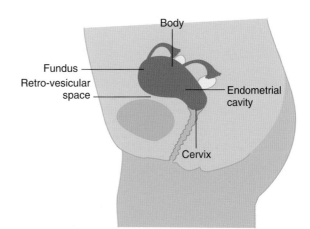

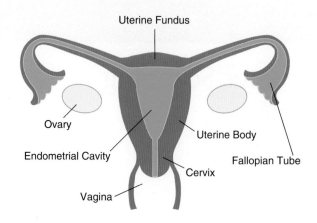

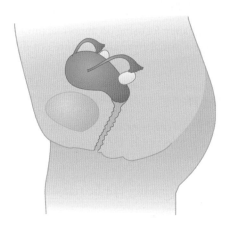

Empty bladder

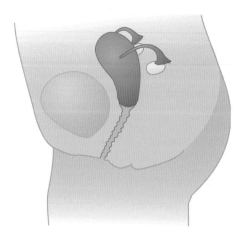

Full Bladder

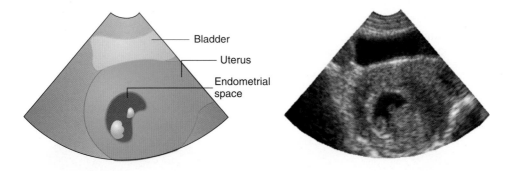

Image Elements

- Contour of uterus
- Endometrial cavity of uterus
- Bladder
- Vaginal stripe

Tricks of the Trade

- Contour and orientation of the uterus are extremely variable from woman to woman and change with volume of urine in the bladder.

- It is helpful to train your eye to search for and identify the long axis view of the uterus to use as a "home base" when imaging the pelvis.

- Probe orientation can be posterior, anterior, left or right due to the orientation of the uterus.

- Filling the bladder results in increased transabdominal views of the uterus and ovaries.

Partial View Probe Positioning

Note: Many of the partial views contain information that is needed to accurately identify pathology. The ideal view may be unobtainable due to patient characteristics and multiple "partial views" will be required to complete the scan.

Too Superior

Bladder on right of screen (if seen)
Limited view of uterus

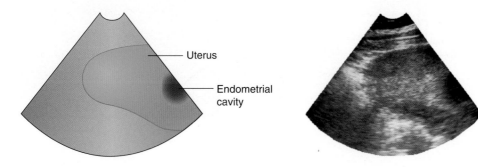

Too Inferior

Uterine fundus not in view
Vaginal stripe centered in view

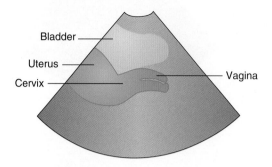

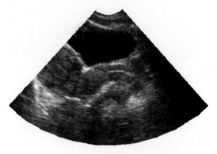

Too Lateral

Uterus off-midline
Endometrial cavity not in view

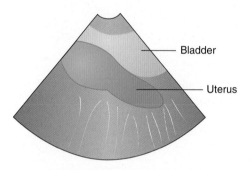

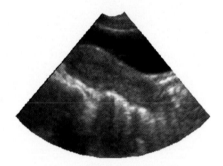

UTERUS LONG AXIS: ENDOVAGINAL

Landmarks

- Bladder
- Uterine outline
- Endometrial stripe/cavity

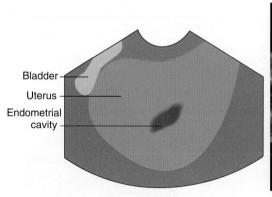

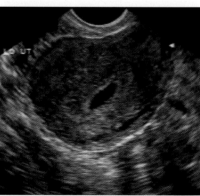

Image Elements

- Contour of uterus
- Endometrial cavity of uterus
- Bladder

Tricks of the Trade

- Emptying the bladder results in improved endovaginal imaging quality.

- It may be necessary to slightly "twist" or rotate the endovaginal probe along its axis in order to observe the entire endometrial stripe.

- It may be necessary to pivot the probe side to side to fully visualize the long axis of the uterus.

- In women who have a very sharply *anteverted* uterus, you may need to pivot the probe so the transducer surface is aimed toward the ceiling.

- In women with *retroverted* uteruses or very full bladders, it may be necessary to pivot the probe so the indicator is toward the floor (aim the transducer surface posteriorly).

- The vesicouterine space is occasionally difficult to image in the sagittal endovaginal route when the bladder is empty.

- It may be necessary to slightly withdraw the probe 1 to 2 centimeters in order to visualize an empty bladder.

Partial View Probe Positioning

Note: Many of the partial views contain information that is needed to accurately identify pathology. The ideal view may be unobtainable due to patient characteristics and multiple "partial views" will be required to complete the scan.

Too Posterior

Uterus on left of screen
Cervix dominates view

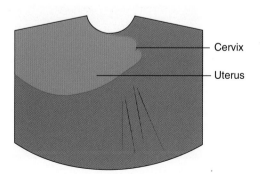

— Cervix
— Uterus

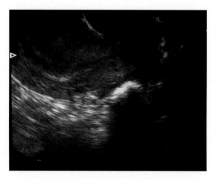

Too Anterior

Bladder dominates view
Uterus on right

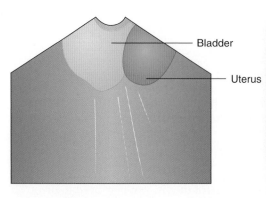

Bladder

Uterus

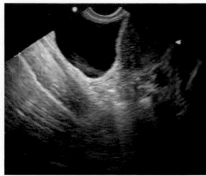

Too Inferior (Probe Not Inserted Enough)

Bladder in view (size depends on volume of urine in bladder)
No or limited uterus seen
Poor image quality

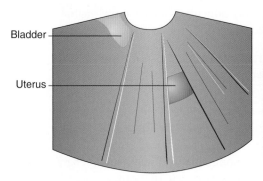

Bladder

Uterus

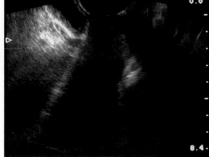

Too Lateral

Uterus off-midline
Endometrial cavity not in view

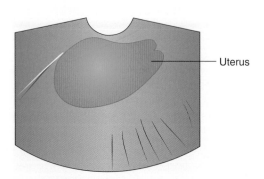

Uterus

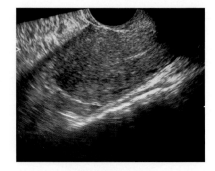

UTERUS SHORT AXIS: TRANSABDOMINAL

Landmarks

- Bladder
- Uterine outline
- Endometrial cavity

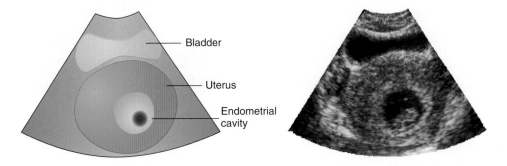

Images

- Contour of uterus
- Endometrial cavity of uterus
- Retrovesicular space

Partial View Probe Positioning

Note: Many of the partial views contain information that is needed to accurately identify pathology. The ideal view may be unobtainable due to patient characteristics and multiple "partial views" will be required to complete the scan.

Too Superior

No bladder or uterus seen, or
Uterus seen but no endometrial cavity seen

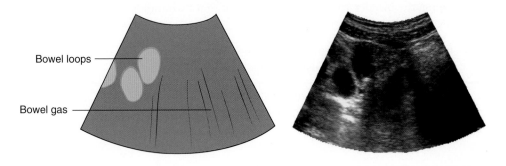

Too Inferior

Pubic symphysis obscures view, or
View of lower uterine segment or cervix

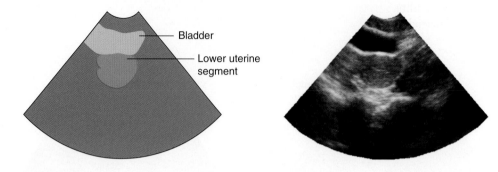

Bladder
Lower uterine segment

Too Lateral

Uterus off-midline

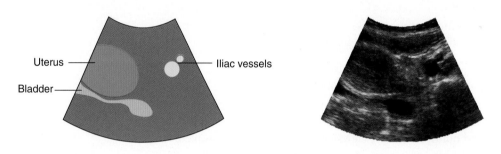

Uterus
Bladder
Iliac vessels

Tricks of the Trade

- Filling the bladder with a Foley catheter or oral hydration will increase image quality during transabdominal imaging.

- It may be necessary to fan very inferiorly in some women who have small uteruses, retroverted uteruses, or larger diameter abdomens.

- In the transverse view, the endometrial "stripe" now appears as the echogenic oval structure at the center of the uterine body.

UTERUS SHORT AXIS: ENDOVAGINAL

Landmarks

- Bladder
- Uterine outline
- Endometrial cavity

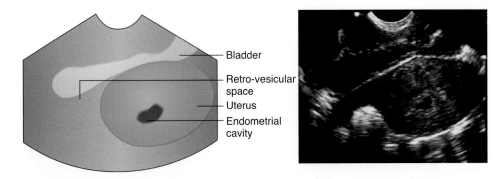

- Bladder
- Retro-vesicular space
- Uterus
- Endometrial cavity

Image Elements

- Contour of uterus
- Endometrial cavity of uterus
- Retrovesicular space

Tricks of the Trade

- The endovaginal coronal plane provides information on the contour of the uterus and may identify pathology not seen on longitudinal plane such as a duplicated or bicornuate uterus.

- It may be necessary to slightly remove the probe 1 to 2 centimeters in order to obtain a view of the retrovesicular space.

- Emptying the bladder will improve image quality during endovaginal imaging.

- Higher imaging quality is obtained with endovaginal imaging than transabdominal imaging.

Partial View Probe Positioning

Note: Many of the partial views contain information that is needed to accurately identify pathology. The ideal view may be unobtainable due to patient characteristics and multiple "partial views" will be required to complete the scan.

Too Posterior

No view of endometrial cavity
Lower uterine segment or cervix dominates view

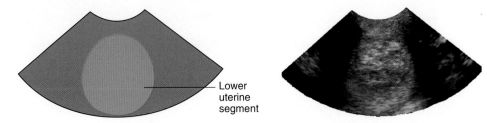

- Lower uterine segment

Too Anterior

Bladder dominates view
No uterus seen

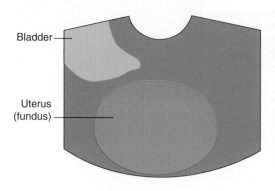

Bladder

Uterus
(fundus)

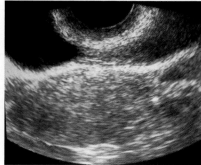

Too Inferior (Probe Not Inserted Far Enough)

Bladder dominates view
No uterus seen

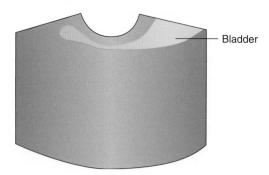

Bladder

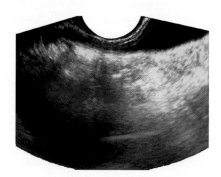

Too Lateral

Uterus off-midline

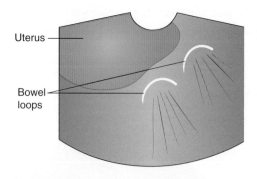

Uterus

Bowel
loops

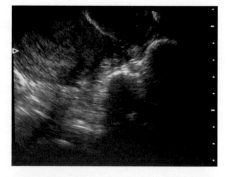

Too Shallow

Incomplete view of uterus and endometrial cavity

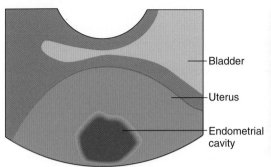
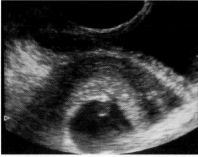

Bladder

Uterus

Endometrial cavity

ADNEXA (RIGHT AND LEFT)

(Note: An additional discussion on imaging the adnexa is contained in Chapter 8 on imaging the ovaries.)

Ovaries and surrounding area may sometimes be seen by transabdominal ultrasound but endovaginal ultrasound is usually required.

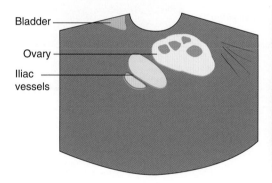
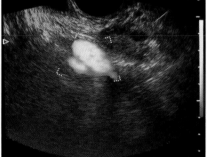

Bladder

Ovary

Iliac vessels

Landmarks

- Iliac artery and vein
- Uterus

Image Elements

- Ovarian silhouette
- Internal ovarian architecture
- Para-ovarian space

Tricks of the Trade

- Finding the ovaries can be an art. Locating them in either sagittal or coronal planes is adequate. Finding the iliac vessel often provides a landmark for locating the ovary. Once the iliac is located, look anterior and medial to locate the ovary.

> • In a transabdominal window, the center of the uterus is the endometrial stripe, or "face of koala bear." To each side of the uterus are the ovaries, or "ears of the koala bear."
>
> • Venous plexus in the adnexa can sometimes look similar to an ovary on gray-scale imaging but will show marked differences with Doppler imaging.
>
> • A normal female will have some small follicular cysts on her ovaries.

UNUSUAL OR ATYPICAL VIEWS

Transabdominal: Uterus On Top of Bladder

- A common normal variant
- Anteroverted and anteroflexed uterus
- Bladder not completely filled

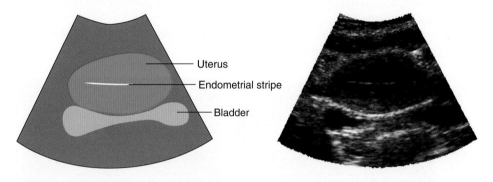

Uterus
Endometrial stripe
Bladder

ULTRASOUND TECHNIQUE

Still Image Protocol

Uterus: Long Axis Transabdominal

Approach – Sagittal anterior
  Transducer infraumbilical, suprapubic
  Mid-abdominal line
  Indicator toward patient's head
  Probe angled toward feet

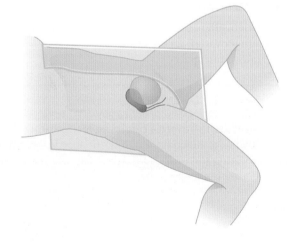

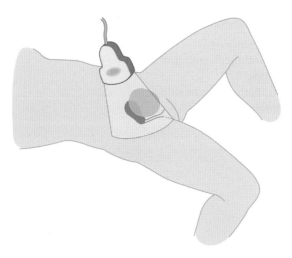

Uterus: Long Axis Endovaginal

Approach – Sagittal inferior
  Transducer intravaginal
  Mid-abdominal line
  Indicator toward ceiling
  Horizontal probe angle is variable, depending on lie of uterus
  Probe handle moved side to side until stripe appears

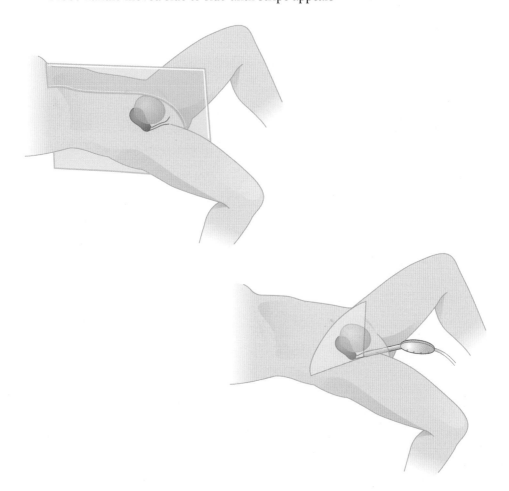

Uterus: Short Axis Transabdominal

Approach – Transverse anterior
  Transducer infraumbilical, suprapubic
  Mid-abdominal line
  Indicator toward patient's right side
  Probe angled toward feet

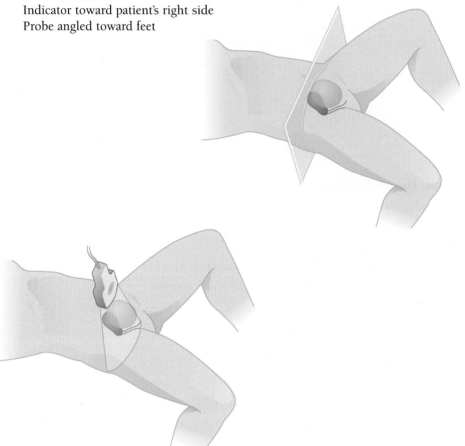

Uterus: Short Axis Endovaginal

Approach – Coronal inferior
 Transducer intravaginal
 Mid-abdominal line
 Indicator toward patient's right leg
 Probe handle lifted toward ceiling or pushed down toward floor

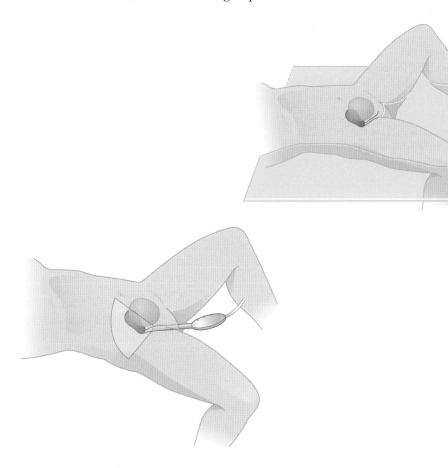

Adnexa: Endovaginal

Approach – Sagittal inferior
 Transducer intravaginal
 Indicator toward ceiling
 Obtain initial view of long axis uterus
 Angle probe laterally
 (+/–) Pivot probe handle toward patient's opposite leg
 Focus on long axis view of iliac vessel
 Focus on ovary silhouette (medial and anterior to iliacs)
 Repeat for opposite side

VIDEOTAPE PROTOCOL

Uterus: Long Axis Transabdominal

Starting point – Sagittal anterior
      Transducer infraumbilical, suprapubic
      Mid-abdominal line
      Indicator toward patient's head
      Probe angled toward feet

Taping protocol
      Focus on longest length of uterus
      Sweep right to left and back
      Include entire length of uterus on screen
      Sweep entire width of uterus
      Focus on uterine cavity
      Sweep entire width of uterine
         cavity

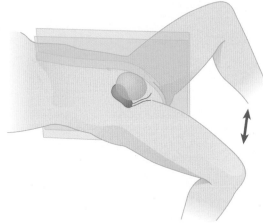

Uterus: Long Axis Endovaginal

Starting point – Sagittal inferior
      Transducer intravaginal
      Orient along mid-abdominal line
      Indicator toward ceiling
      Horizontal orientation variable, slight angle down or horizontal

Taping protocol
      Focus on longest axis of uterus
      Sweep left to right and back
      Include entire length of uterus
         on screen
      Sweep entire width of uterus
      Focus on endometrial cavity
      Sweep entire width of cavity

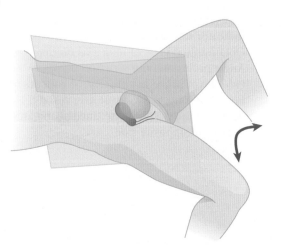

Uterus: Transabdominal Short Axis

Starting point – Transverse anterior
    Transducer infraumbilical, suprapubic
    Mid-abdominal line
    Indicator toward patient's right side
    Probe angled toward feet

Taping protocol
    Focus on outline of uterus
    Sweep superior to inferior and back
    Include entire width of uterus on screen
    Sweep entire length of uterus
    Focus on uterine cavity
    Sweep entire length of uterine cavity

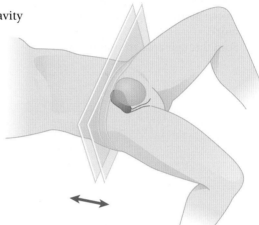

Uterus: Endovaginal Short Axis

Starting point – Transverse inferior
    Transducer endovaginal
    Mid-abdominal line
    Indicator toward ceiling
    Probe angled toward floor

Taping protocol
    Focus on outline of uterus
    Sweep anterior to posterior and back
    Include entire width of uterus on screen
    Sweep entire length of uterus
    Focus on uterine cavity
    Sweep entire length of uterine
        cavity

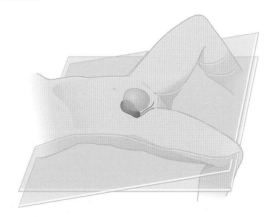

Adnexa: Endovaginal

Starting point – Sagittal inferior
  Transducer endovaginal
  Indicator toward ceiling
  Obtain initial view of long axis uterus
  Angle probe laterally
  (+/–) Pivot probe handle toward patient's opposite leg
  Focus on long axis view of iliac vessel
  Focus on ovary silhouette (medial and anterior to iliacs)
  Repeat for opposite side

Taping protocol
  Focus on outline of ovary
  Sweep probe medial–lateral or obliquely anterior superior (perpendicular to probe indicator)
  Scan through area around ovary

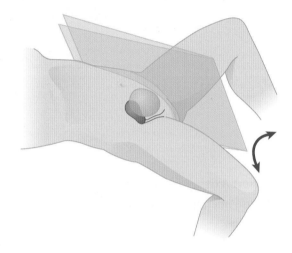

Ovarian Scanning Protocol

J. Christian Fox

GOAL OF AN OVARIAN ULTRASOUND

Demonstrate abnormalities in the ovary focusing on abnormal ovarian architecture (cysts, masses) or blood flow to ovary.

EMERGENCY ULTRASOUND APPROACH

Emergency medicine ultrasound of the ovary is focused on the clinical questions involving possible abnormalities of the ovary. Patients with pelvic pain are commonly seen in the emergency department. The most common yes–no questions addressed for these patients are those pertaining to ovarian cysts (i.e., ruptured, hemorrhagic). The most serious yes–no question involving the ovary is the question of ovarian torsion.

There are two diagnostic approaches for patients with a concern of ovarian torsion. One is to look for alternative diagnoses that will explain the patient's symptoms; the other is to look for ovarian torsion directly. In either case additional imaging is required if the emergency ultrasound does not provide a conclusive diagnosis. Directly imaging the ovary and paraovarian space may provide all of the information that is needed for a diagnosis. Doppler imaging may demonstrate decreased blood flow consistent with ovarian torsion. Indirect information on ovarian pathology can be gathered by demonstrating fluid in the dependent portion of the pelvis (i.e., pouch of Douglas or retrovesicular pouch).

Doppler ultrasound can provide useful information during the evaluation of the ovary. It is used to evaluate blood flow to the ovaries. However, Doppler ultrasound is an advanced technique that can be difficult to master. Some physicians may not feel comfortable mastering Doppler imaging. Conditions such as ovarian torsion may intermittently demonstrate normal blood flow and decreased blood flow may be seen in a normal ovary. A complete discussion of Doppler ultrasound is beyond the scope of this book. As with all emergency ultrasound protocols, gray-scale imaging is critical prior to beginning any Doppler assessment.

ANATOMY

The anatomy of interest involves the ovary and surrounding tissues. The ovary has a somewhat variable location within the female pelvis. The ovaries are found anterior and medial to the iliac vessels and measure $2 \times 2 \times 3$ centimeters.

Ovary
    Left
    Right
Uterus
Iliac artery
Iliac vein
Retrovesicular space
Pouch of Douglas

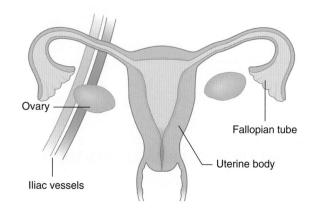

PATIENT POSITION

Supine
Thighs abducted

PATIENT PREPARATION

- Endovaginal – Empty bladder improves imaging of uterus and ovaries
- Transabdominal – Full bladder improves images of uterus but usually has no effect on imaging ovaries

TRANSDUCER

Endovaginal – 5 to 7.5 MHz
Transabdominal – 3 to 5 MHz

OVARIAN PATHOLOGY

- Masses within the ovary can represent neoplastic activity
  (Note: Ovarian neoplasms vary in ultrasonographic appearance and a full description is beyond the scope of this book.)
- Ovarian cysts (anechoic structures) within the ovary can represent normal follicular rupture, hemorrhagic cysts, or simple cysts
- Complex fluid collections in the adnexa can represent infection or ectopic pregnancy
- Free fluid in the pelvis may be a nonspecific sign of pathology in the pelvis

OVARY ESSENTIAL IMAGES

- Right ovary
  - Sagittal view
  - Coronal view
  - Doppler images
- Left ovary
  - Sagittal view
  - Coronal view
  - Doppler images
- Inferior pelvic recess
  - Pouch of Douglas
  - Retrovesicular pouch

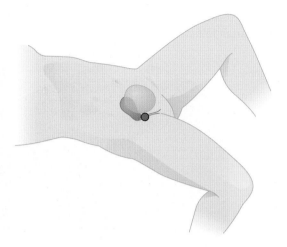

Tricks of the Trade

- In women who are multiparous, the ovaries have a more variable location. Occasionally they are located more anterior. Attempting to visualize anterior ovaries using the endovaginal probe can cause discomfort or not be possible at all. Therefore it may be necessary to use the transabdominal approach in these women.

- It is common for the novice sonographer to mistake bowel for ovary. Recall that bowel regularly demonstrates peristalsis and readily slides when pressure is applied with the probe.

- A normal female will have some small follicular cysts on her ovaries.

- Set the initial color/power Doppler gain, filter, pulse repetition frequency (PRF), and scale low enough so you can identify slow velocities within the ovary.

ENDOVAGINAL OVARY

Note: In normal patient anatomy, left and right ovarian images are nearly identical. Landmarks, image elements, and poor probe positions are unchanged. Labeling as left or right ovary is crucial for later interpretation.

Ovary: Endovaginal, Sagittal
Landmarks
- Iliac vessels
- Ovarian follicles

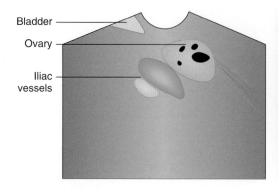
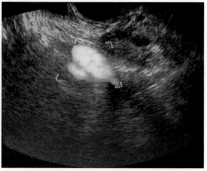

Bladder ——

Ovary —

Iliac
vessels ——

(Note: Doppler imaging is not needed to find the ovary in most patients.)

Image Elements
- Ovary
- Paraovarian space

Image Characteristics
- Ovary contour
- Ovary internal architecture
  - Small internal cysts
- Ovary with color and spectral Doppler (both venous and arterial)

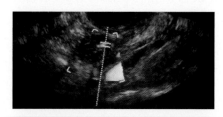

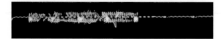

Ovarian Venous Waveform

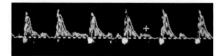

Ovarian Arterial Waveform

Tricks of the Trade

- Finding the ovary can be an art. Imaging the adnexa in a sagittal plane will result in a long axis view of the iliac vessels. The ovary should lie just medial and anterior to the iliac vessels.

- It may be necessary to gently insert the endovaginal probe further in order to visualize the ovaries.

- Pelvic structures such as the ovary, fallopian tube, and bowel should all slide easily among one another when pressure is applied with the probe. This "sliding organ sign" helps to rule out pathology.

- Elevating the pelvis off the stretcher as in a speculum examination allows for a full range of movement of the endovaginal probe.

- Endovaginal imaging of the ovaries is superior to transabdominal imaging.

- Pelvic vessels can mimic the appearance of an ovary with follicular cysts. The short axis of these vessels may appear as cysts (round, anechoic) but the vessels will elongate with probe rotation. Doppler can also be used to differentiate uterine vasculature from ovarian follicles.

Partial View Probe Positioning

Note: Many of the partial views contain information that is needed to accurately identify pathology. The ideal view may be unobtainable due to patient characteristics and multiple "partial views" will be required to complete the scan.

Too Medial

Uterus dominates view
No view of ovary

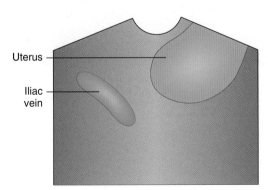
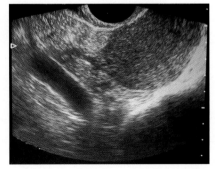

Too Anterior, Posterior, or Lateral

Bowel or soft tissue dominates view
No view of ovary

OVARY: ENDOVAGINAL CORONAL

Landmarks

- Uterus (+/–)
- Ovarian follicles

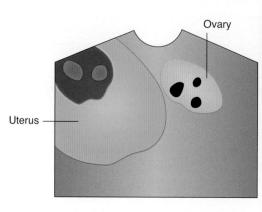
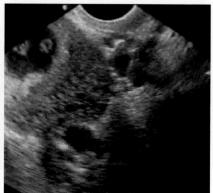

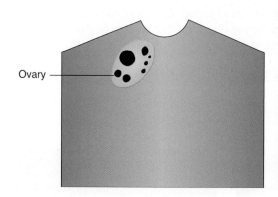
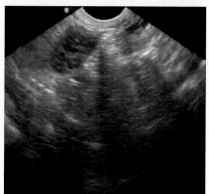

Image Elements

- Ovary
- Paraovarian space

Image Characteristics

- Ovary contour
- Ovary internal architecture
  - Small internal cysts

Tricks of the Trade

- Doppler imaging does not need to be obtained in more than one plane.

- When attempting to locate the ovaries it is easy to get "lost." Re-center probe on coronal view of uterus and advance laterally to adnexa or find ovary in sagittal axis and rotate 90 degrees.

Partial View Probe Positioning

Note: Many of the partial views contain information that is needed to accurately identify pathology. The ideal view may be unobtainable due to patient characteristics and multiple "partial views" will be required to complete the scan.

Too Medial

Uterus dominates view
No view of ovary

Too Anterior, Posterior, or Lateral

Bowel dominates view
No view of ovary

OVARY: TRANSABDOMINAL

Imaging the ovaries using a transabdominal approach is difficult. Superior views are achieved using an endovaginal approach.

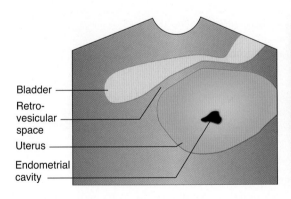
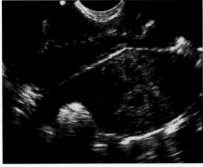

Bladder
Retro-vesicular space
Uterus
Endometrial cavity

OVARY: TRANSABDOMINAL, SAGITTAL

Landmarks

- Ovarian silhouette

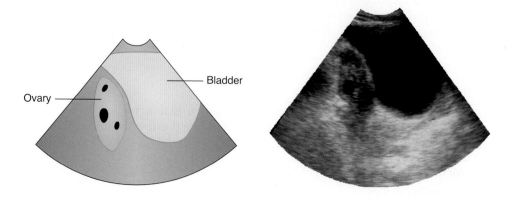

Image Elements

- Ovary
- Bladder

Image Characteristics

- Ovarian contour
- Ovarian internal architecture

Tricks of the Trade

- A full bladder will greatly improve image quality.

- If unable to visualize the ovary transabdominally, drain the bladder and image the ovary endovaginally.

- Doppler imaging of the ovary is better performed during endovaginal ultrasound.

Partial View Probe Positioning

Most partial views of the ovary are images where the ovary is not centered in the screen. Atypical probe positions during a transabdominal ultrasound of the ovary will result in no visualization of the ovary.

OVARY: TRANSABDOMINAL, TRANSVERSE

Landmarks

- Uterine body
- (+/−) Iliac vessels

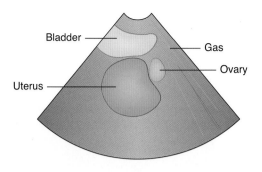 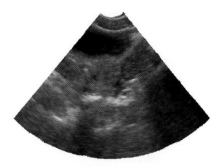

Image Elements

- Ovary contour
- Ovary internal architecture
- Ovary with Doppler

Tricks of the Trade

- Applying firm pressure with the transducer will displace tissue and bowel resulting in improved image quality but may cause the patient some discomfort if the bladder is full.

- In a transabdominal window, the center of the uterus is the endometrial stripe, or "face of koala bear." To each side of the uterus are the ovaries, or "ears of the koala bear."

Partial View Probe Positioning

Many partial views of the ovary are images where the ovary is not centered in the screen. Atypical probe positions during a transabdominal ultrasound of the ovary will result in no visualization of the ovary.

Too Superior or Inferior

No view of ovary
Uterus in view

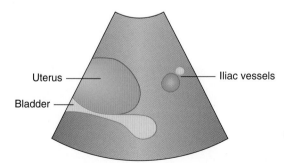 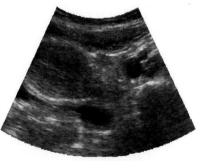

Too Lateral

Bowel dominates view
No view of ovary

PELVIC CUL-DE-SACS

Landmarks

- Bladder
- Uterus

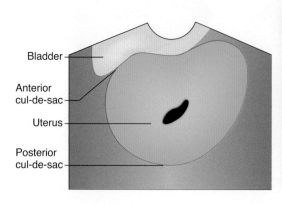
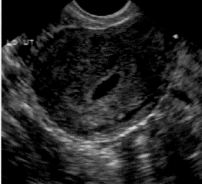

Image Elements

- Contour of uterus
- Contour of bladder
- Anterior cul-de-sac, *or*, rectouterine space
- Posterior cul-de-sac, *or*, vesicouterine space, *or*, pouch of Douglas

---

Tricks of the Trade

- A small amount of fluid in the rectouterine space (posterior cul-de-sac) is normal.

- Fluid in the vesicouterine pouch (anterior cul-de-sac) is almost never normal and should arouse suspicion of a pathologic condition.

Partial View Probe Positioning
Too Lateral

Bladder small or not seen
Limited view of recesses

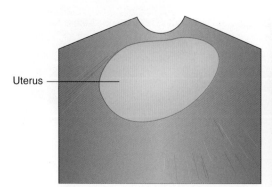
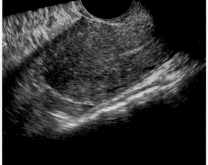

Too Inferior

Poor image quality, *or*
Bladder dominates view
No view of pouch of Douglas

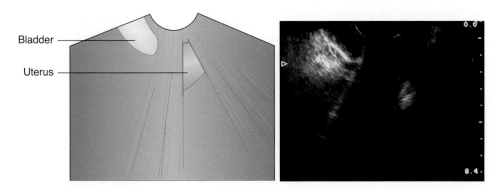

Too Anterior

Bladder dominates view
Uterus on right of image
Limited view of posterior cul-de-sac

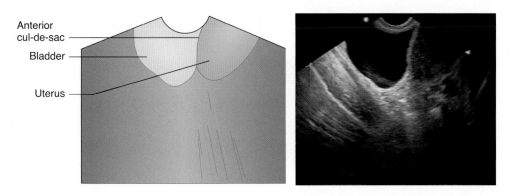

Too Posterior

Uterus dominates view
Limited or no view of anterior cul-de-sac

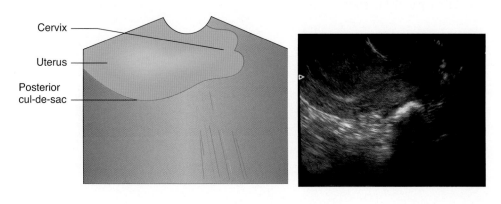

ULTRASOUND TECHNIQUE

Still Image Protocol

Left Ovary: Sagittal

Approach – Sagittal, inferior
    Transducer – Endovaginal
    Orient probe toward left shoulder
    Indicator toward ceiling
    Probe parallel to stretcher

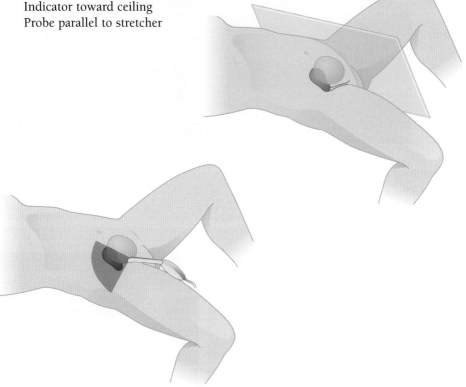

Right Ovary: Sagittal

Approach – Sagittal, inferior
    Transducer – Endovaginal
    Orient probe toward right shoulder
    Indicator toward ceiling
    Probe parallel to stretcher

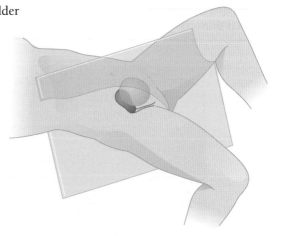

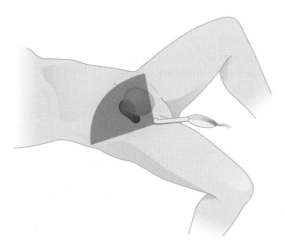

Left Ovary: Coronal

Approach – Coronal, inferior
 Transducer – Endovaginal
  Orient probe toward left shoulder
  Indicator toward patient's right
  Probe parallel to stretcher

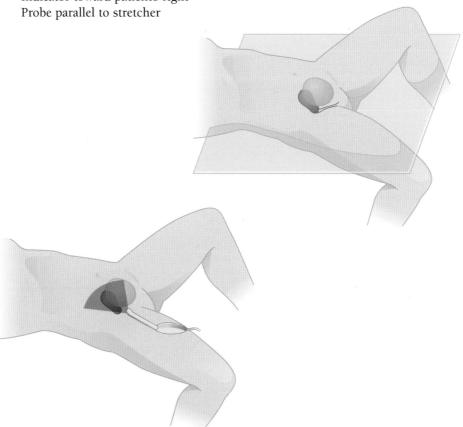

Right Ovary: Coronal

Approach – Coronal, inferior
    Transducer – Endovaginal
      Orient probe toward right shoulder
      Indicator toward patient's left
      Probe parallel to stretcher

Pelvic Recess (Anterior and Posterior Cul-de-sac)

Approach – Sagittal, inferior
    Transducer – Endovaginal
      Mid-abdominal line
      Indicator toward ceiling
      Probe oriented slightly toward
        floor

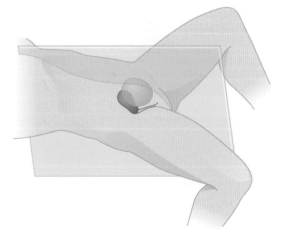

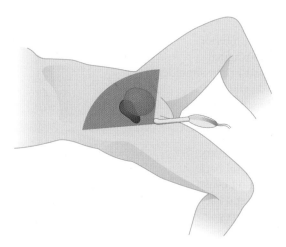

VIDEOTAPE PROTOCOL

Ovary: Left

Starting point – Sagittal, inferior
    Transducer – Endovaginal
    Orient probe toward left shoulder
    Indicator toward ceiling
    Probe parallel to stretcher

Taping protocol
    Focus on long axis of ovary
    Sweep right to left and back
    Focus on area around ovary
    Sweep left to right and back
    Rotate probe 90 degrees
        counterclockwise
    Move handle up and down

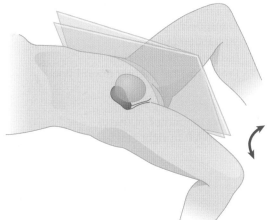

Ovary: Right

Starting point – Sagittal, inferior
> Transducer – Endovaginal
> Orient probe toward right shoulder
> Indicator toward ceiling
> Probe parallel to stretcher

Taping protocol
> Focus on long axis of ovary
> Sweep right to left and back
> Focus on area around ovary
> Sweep left to right and back
> Rotate probe 90 degrees
>> clockwise
> Move handle up and down

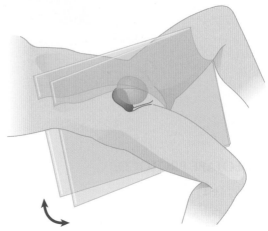

Pelvic Recess (Anterior and Posterior Cul-de-Sac)

Starting point – Sagittal, inferior
> Transducer – Endovaginal
> Mid-abdominal line
> Indicator toward ceiling
> Probe oriented slightly toward floor

Taping protocol
> Focus on outline of uterus
> Sweep left to right and back

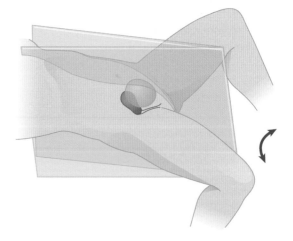

VASCULAR PROTOCOLS

Aorta Scanning Protocol

Romolo Gaspari

GOAL OF AORTA ULTRASOUND

Demonstrate abnormalities in abdominal aorta primarily related to size.

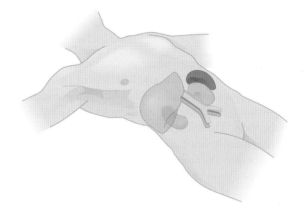

EMERGENCY ULTRASOUND APPROACH

Emergency ultrasound of the aorta is focused on the clinical questions involving the abdominal aorta. Patients with back pain, abdominal pain, or flank pain are commonly seen in the emergency department. The most common yes–no questions addressed with an emergency medicine ultrasound of the abdominal aorta are those pertaining to aneurysmal dilatation of the aorta.

ANATOMY

The anatomy of interest in the aorta scan involves the abdominal aorta and the area around the aorta.
Aorta
    Upper aorta
    Middle aorta
    Lower aorta

Prevertebral space
Celiac artery
    Hepatic artery
    Splenic artery
    Left gastric artery
Superior mesenteric artery (SMA)
Iliac arteries
Inferior vena cava
Splenic vein
Left renal vein

The aorta follows the natural curvature of the spine in its course through the abdomen, lying immediately anterior and slightly left of the spine. The prevertebral space is the area between the shadow of the lumbar spine and the aorta. The upper aorta consists of the portion containing the first two sonographically identified arteries: the celiac artery and the SMA. The middle aorta consists of the portion of the aorta with no sonographically recognizable branches. The inferior aorta consists of the portion where the aorta bifurcates into the iliac arteries just under the umbilicus. The inferior vena cava runs roughly parallel to the aorta, along the right side of the spine.

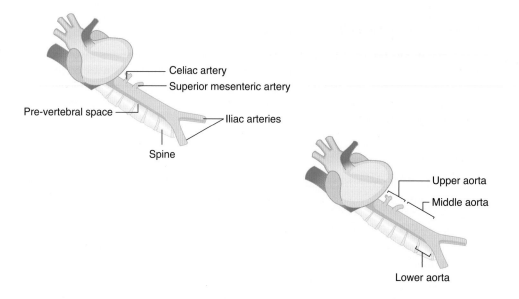

The celiac artery (or celiac trunk) is the first major branch of the abdominal aorta and runs perpendicular to the aorta. This is a short vessel that quickly branches into the splenic and hepatic arteries (which are commonly seen) and the left gastric artery (which is not). In a transverse window, the celiac, hepatic, and splenic arteries form the shape of a mustache, seagull, or the letter T. The body of the seagull is the celiac artery with the right and left wings formed by the hepatic and splenic arteries. The second branch of the abdominal aorta, the SMA, courses parallel to the aorta inferiorly. In a short axis the SMA appears as a "mantle clock" or a white triangle with a dark circular center due to the hyperechoic fat and muscle surrounding the vessel as it exits the aorta.

PATIENT POSITION

Supine

PATIENT PREPARATION

Not applicable

TRANSDUCER

2.5 to 5.0 MHz curved or phased array probe

AORTA PATHOLOGY

- Aortic dissection and atherosclerosis result in intraluminal echoes
- Aortic aneurysms result in dilatation of aorta
- Leaking aortic aneurysms rarely show free abdominal fluid

ULTRASOUND IMAGES

Aorta Essential Images

- Aorta long axis
  - Superior aorta
  - Middle aorta
  - Inferior aorta
- Aorta short or transverse axis
  - Superior aorta
  - Middle aorta
  - Inferior aorta

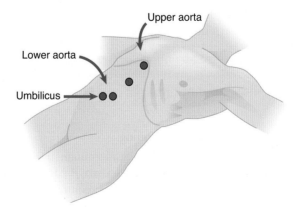

> *Tricks of the Trade*
>
> - Gentle persistent pressure helps displace bowel loops to improve visualization of the abdominal aorta.
>
> - Occasionally firm pressure is necessary in larger patients, or those with large amounts of bowel gas.

AORTA LONGITUDINAL, SUPERIOR

Landmarks

- Spinal shadow
- Celiac artery
- SMA

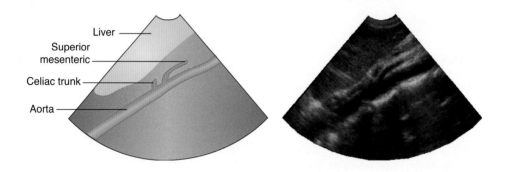

Image Elements

- Aorta contour
- Aorta internal architecture

> *Tricks of the Trade*
>
> - Superior views of the aorta can be easily distinguished from the superior vena cava by looking for the celiac or superior mesenteric arteries.
>
> - Bowel gas from the stomach that is obscuring your view may be decreased by turning the patient onto the right lateral decubitus to pool fluid in the stomach into the antrum.
>
> - Longer length of time spent performing ultrasound of the abdomen will increase the amount of bowel activity and bowel gas, thereby decreasing image quality.

Partial View Probe Positioning

Note: Many of the partial views contain information that is needed to accurately identify pathology. The ideal view may be unobtainable due to patient characteristics and multiple "partial views" will be required to complete the scan.

Too Superior

Liver and cardiac structures dominate view
Images are short axis, subxiphoid views
No aorta in view

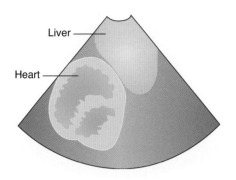

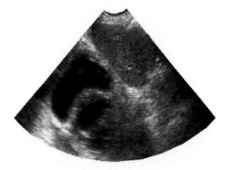

Too Caudal

Aorta in view
No celiac artery or SMA
Images are mid-aorta or lower aorta views

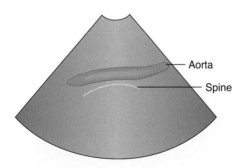

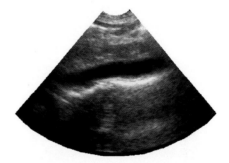

Too Lateral Right

Inferior vena cava (IVC) dominates view

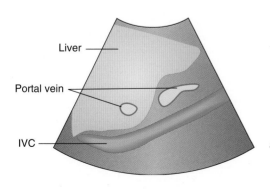

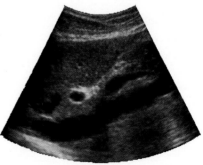

Too Lateral Left

Bowel loops dominate view, *or*
Stomach dominates view
Poor image quality

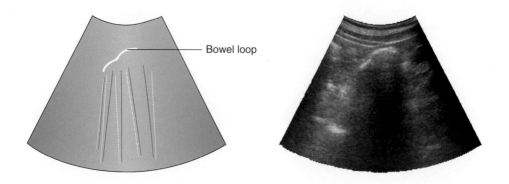

Aorta longitudinal, middle

Landmarks

- Spinal shadow
- Liver (+/–)

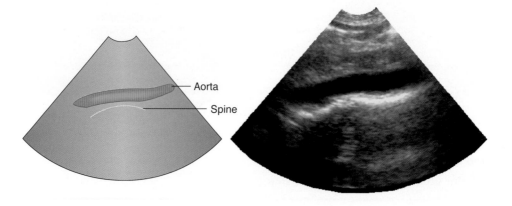

Image Elements

- Aorta contour
- Aorta internal architecture

Tricks of the Trade

- Slow, steady pressure on the ultrasound probe will displace bowel loops and increase image quality.

- The aorta follows the lumbar lordosis and courses from "deep to shallow," while the IVC has a more level course in the abdomen.

- An ectatic aorta may follow an abnormal path in the abdomen; if you lose the aorta, go back to where you initially saw it (long or transverse).

Partial View Probe Positioning

Note: Many of the partial views contain information that is needed to accurately identify pathology. The ideal view may be unobtainable due to patient characteristics and multiple "partial views" will be required to complete the scan.

Too Superior

Celiac artery and SMA in view
View is of superior aorta

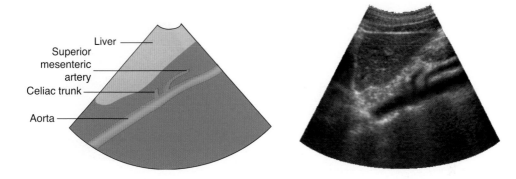

Too Caudal

Iliac artery in view
Looks very similar to middle aorta in longitudinal plane (but probe is inferior to umbilicus)

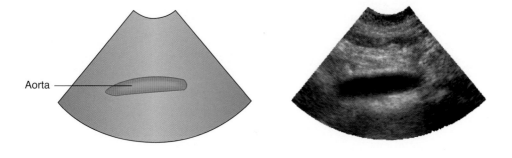

Too Lateral Left

Bowel loops dominate view
May see lower edge of spleen
May see left kidney

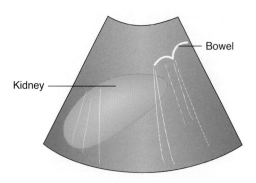
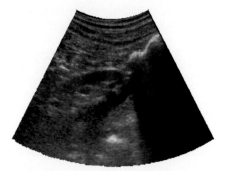

Too Lateral Right

IVC in view
Looks similar to middle aorta

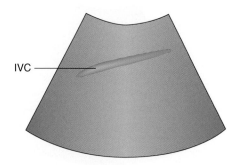
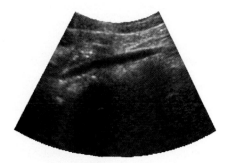

Tricks of the Trade

- If you are unsure the vascular structure is vena cava or aorta, scan laterally and medially to identify other vascular structures, *or*

- Return to superior aorta, identify celiac or superior mesenteric artery and trace inferiorly, *or*

- Rotate probe to transverse view and identify spinal shadow, *or*

- Use Doppler signal to identify arterial waveform.

AORTA LONGITUDINAL, LOW

Landmarks

- Spinal shadow

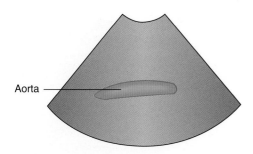
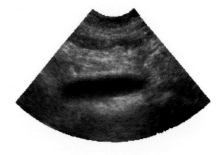

Image Elements

- Aorta contour
- Aorta internal architecture

Partial View Probe Positioning

Note: Many of the partial views contain information that is needed to accurately identify pathology. The ideal view may be unobtainable due to patient characteristics and multiple "partial views" will be required to complete the scan.

Too Superior

Middle aorta in view
Looks almost identical to lower aorta

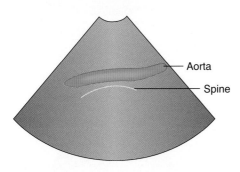
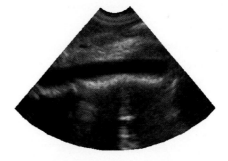

Too Caudal

Iliac vessel in view, *or*
Bowel loops dominate view
Poor image quality

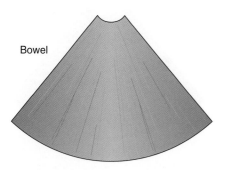

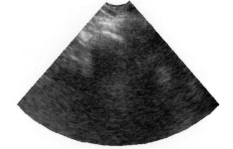

Too Lateral Right

IVC in view

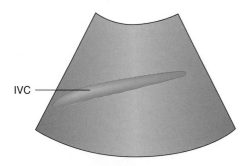

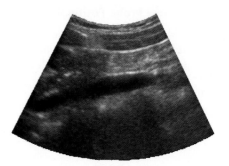

Too Lateral Left

Bowel loops dominate view
Poor image quality

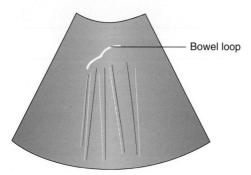

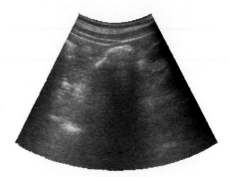

Tricks of the Trade

- When sliding probe inferiorly in long axis, differentiating distal aorta from proximal iliac is difficult to determine from long axis ultrasound images.

- If image of aorta is lost in bowel gas while sliding inferiorly, return to previously identified segment and retrace inferiorly.

- A quick transverse view will demonstrate the iliac bifurcation in cases where the long axis view is not definitive.

AORTA TRANSVERSE, SUPERIOR

Landmarks

- Spinal shadow
- Celiac artery
- SMA

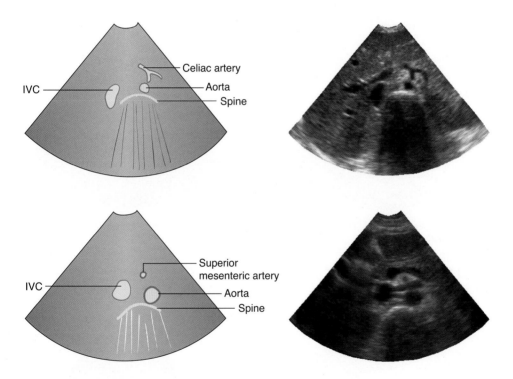

Image Elements

- Aorta contour
- Aorta internal architecture

Partial View Probe Positioning

Note: Many of the partial views contain information that is needed to accurately identify pathology. The ideal view may be unobtainable due to patient characteristics and multiple "partial views" will be required to complete the scan.

Too Caudal

Aorta in view
No celiac artery or superior mesenteric artery
Image is view of middle aorta

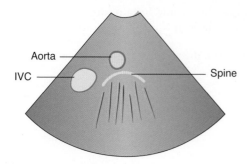
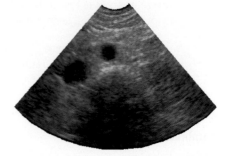

Too Lateral Right

Aorta off center
IVC centered in view

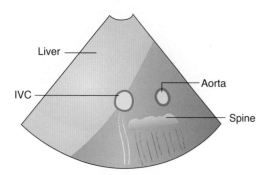
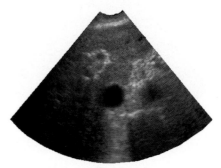

Too Lateral Left

Aorta off center
Bowel loops dominate view
Stomach gas obscured aorta

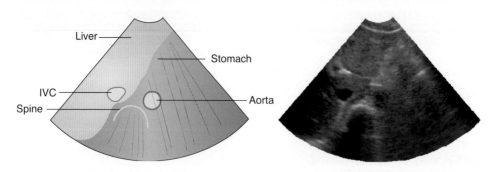

AORTA TRANSVERSE, MIDDLE

Landmarks

- Spinal shadow

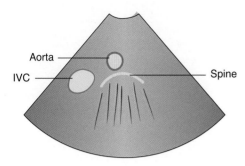

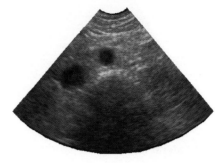

Images

- Aorta contour
- Aorta internal architecture

Tricks of the Trade

- Anterior–posterior measurement of the aorta for dilatation can be artificially increased if the ultrasound probe is held perpendicular to the abdominal wall due to the lumbar lordosis of the aorta. The ultrasound probe should be angled 5 to 10 degrees cephalad for more accurate measurements.

Partial View Probe Positioning

Note: Many of the partial views contain information that is needed to accurately identify pathology. The ideal view may be unobtainable due to patient characteristics and multiple "partial views" will be required to complete the scan.

Too Superior

Celiac artery in view, or
SMA in view
View is of superior aorta

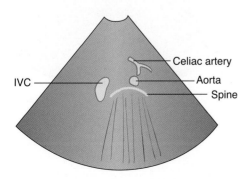

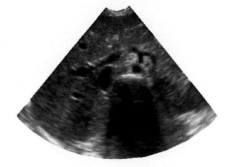

Too Caudal

View is of distal aorta or iliacs

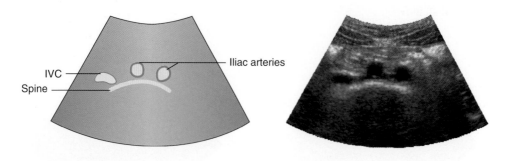

Too Lateral Right

Aorta off center
IVC centered in view

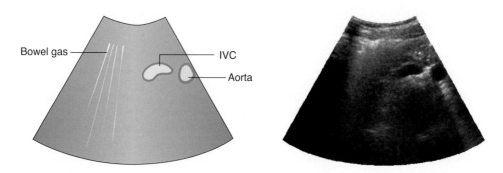

Too Lateral Left

Aorta off center
Bowel loops dominate view

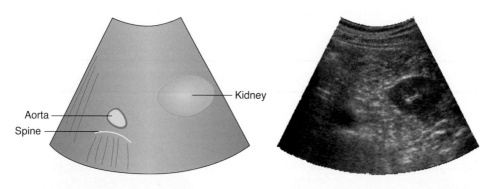

AORTA TRANSVERSE, LOW

Landmarks

- Spinal shadow
- Iliac bifurcation

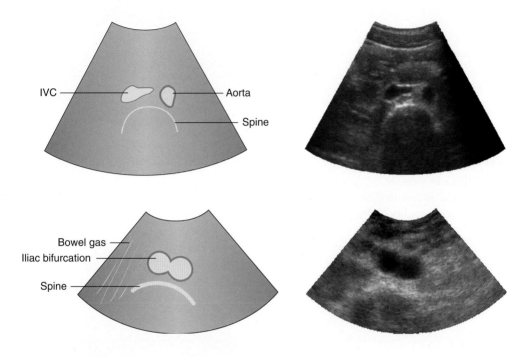

Image Elements

- Aorta contour
- Aorta internal architecture

Tricks of the Trade

- Avoid imaging aorta or iliac bifurcation directly over umbilicus as air is commonly trapped there and can degrade the image quality.

- Include views of iliac bifurcation in lower aorta views as pathology may sometimes be only seen at iliac/aorta junction.

- Inferior aorta is closest to abdominal wall (and ultrasound probe) due to lumbar lordosis.

Partial View Probe Positioning

Note: Many of the partial views contain information that is needed to accurately identify pathology. The ideal view may be unobtainable due to patient characteristics and multiple "partial views" will be required to complete the scan.

Too Superior

Middle aorta in view

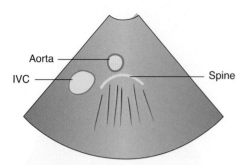
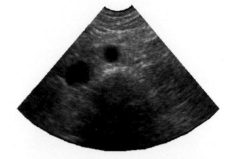

Too Caudal

Distal iliacs in view, *or*
Bowel loops dominate view
Usually image quality is degraded

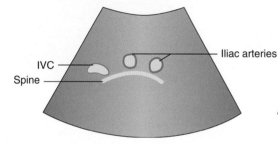
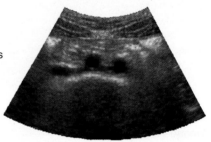

Too Lateral Right

Proximal iliacs or aorta off center to right
IVC centered in view, *or*
Bowel loops dominate view

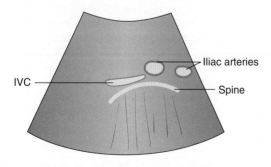
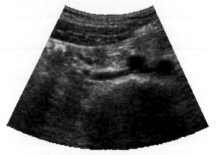

Too Lateral Left

Proximal iliacs off center to left, *or*
Bowel loops dominate view

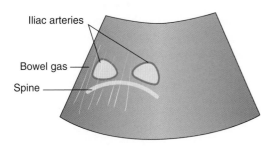

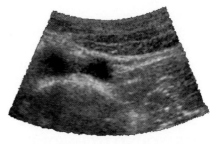

Alternative Views

Coronal view of aorta and vena cava

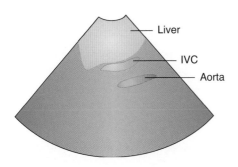

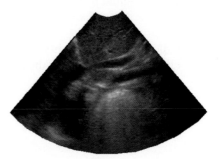

IVC centered in view, mistaken for aorta
Lack of spinal shadow

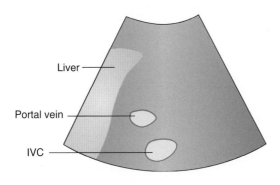

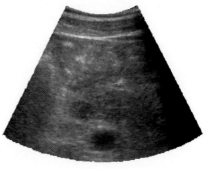

AORTA VS. VENA CAVA

Mistaking the vena cava for the aorta is a common error of novice ultrasonographers. Some aspects of the images that differentiate one from the other are as follows:

	Aorta	Vena Cava
Pulsations	Single strong pulsation	Double wavy pulsation
Course in abdomen	"Deep to shallow"	Parallel to abdominal wall
Vessels seen on ultrasound	SMA and celiac	None
Transverse silhouette	Round	Variable
Location to spine	Directly anterior	Right lateral
Changes with inspiration	None	Increase diameter

ULTRASOUND TECHNIQUE

Still Image Protocol

Aorta: Long Axis, Superior

Approach – Sagittal plane, anterior
 Transducer at subxiphoid
 Epigastrium
 Indicator toward patient's head
 Probe perpendicular to skin

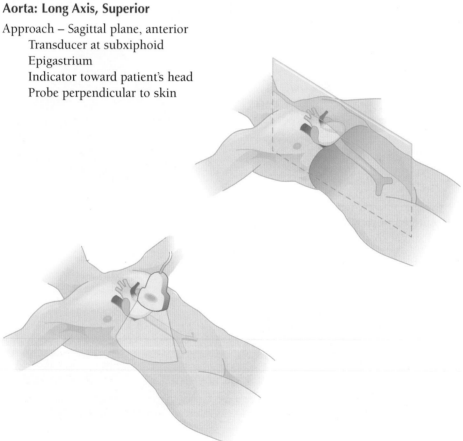

Aorta: Long Axis, Mid

Approach – Sagittal plane, anterior

    Transducer halfway from epigastrium to umbilicus

    Mid-abdominal line

    Indicator toward patient's head

    Probe perpendicular to skin or angled toward head

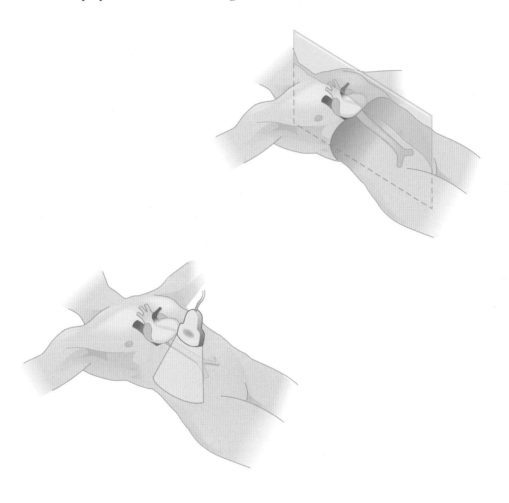

Aorta: Long Axis, Low

Approach – Sagittal plane, anterior
  Transducer halfway from epigastrium to umbilicus
  Mid-abdominal line
  Indicator toward patient's head
  Probe perpendicular to skin or angled toward head

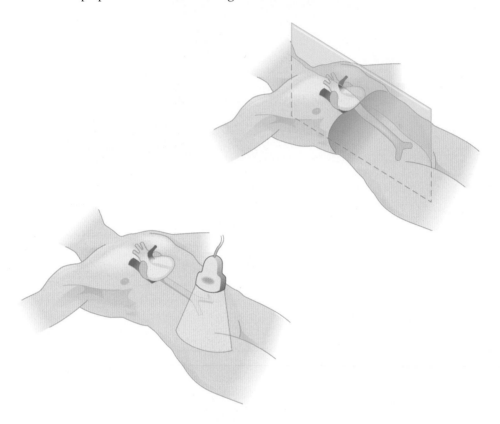

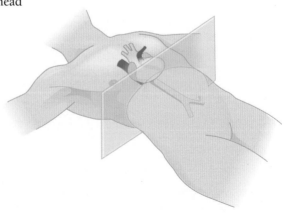

Aorta: Transverse or Short Axis, Superior

Approach – Transverse plane, anterior
  Transducer at subxiphoid
  Epigastrium
  Indicator toward patient's right side
  Angle probe slightly toward head

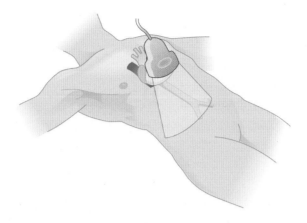

Aorta: Short or Transverse Axis, Mid

Approach – Transverse plane, anterior
    Transducer halfway from epigastrium to umbilicus
    Mid-abdominal line
    Indicator toward patient's right side
    Angle probe slightly toward head

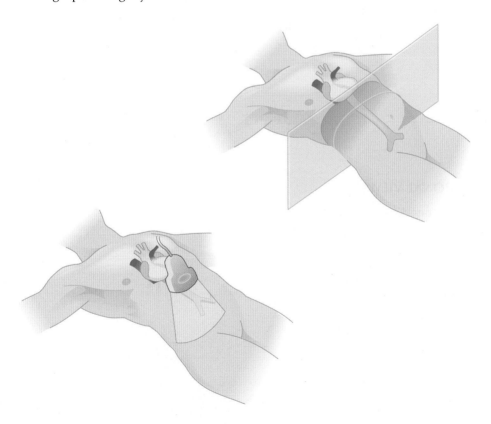

Aorta: Short or Transverse Axis, Low

Approach – Transverse plane, anterior
    Transducer periumbilical
    Mid-abdominal line
    Indicator toward patient's right side
    Angle probe slightly toward head

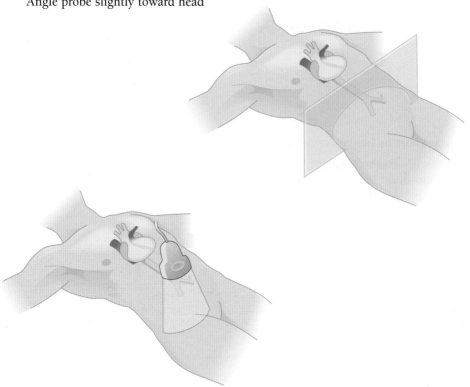

OPTIONAL VIEWS

Aorta: Long Axis, Coronal

Approach – Coronal plane, lateral
    Transducer at costal margin
    Mid-axillary line
    Indicator toward patient's head
    Probe perpendicular to skin

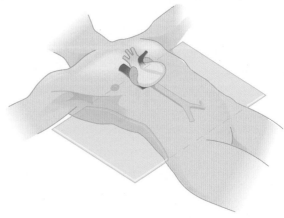

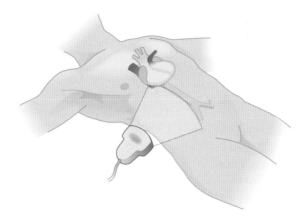

VIDEOTAPE PROTOCOL

Aorta: Long Axis

Starting point – Sagittal plane, anterior
    Transducer at epigastrium
    Mid-abdominal line (line from subxiphoid to umbilicus)
    Indicator toward patient's head
    Probe perpendicular to skin

Taping protocol
    Focus on area anterior to spine
    Sweep superior to inferior
    Follow course of aorta
    Include entire length of aorta

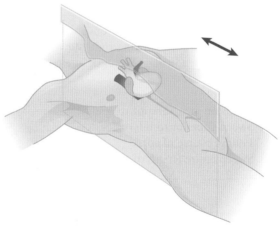

–Alternative–

Starting point – Coronal plane, transverse
>   Transducer at costal margin
>   Right middle axillary line
>   Indicator toward patient's head
>   Probe perpendicular to skin

Taping protocol
>   Focus on aorta silhouette
>   Sweep superior to inferior
>   Follow course of aorta
>   Sweep entire length of aorta

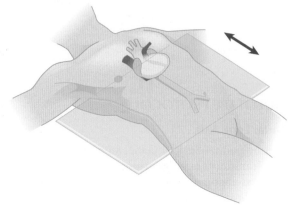

Aorta: Short Axis

Starting point – Transverse plane, anterior
>   Transducer at epigastrium
>   Mid-abdominal line (line from subxiphoid to umbilicus)
>   Indicator toward patient's right side
>   Probe perpendicular to skin or angled slightly toward head

Taping protocol
>   Focus on area anterior to spine
>   Sweep superior to inferior
>   Follow course of aorta
>   Sweep entire length of aorta

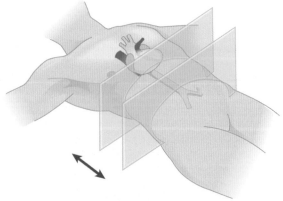

Lower Extremity Vascular Scanning Protocol

J. Christian Fox

GOAL OF LOWER EXTREMITY VASCULAR ULTRASOUND

Demonstrate abnormalities in the veins of the leg primarily related to obstruction of venous flow.

EMERGENCY ULTRASOUND APPROACH

Emergency medicine lower extremity vascular ultrasound is focused on the clinical questions involving pain and swelling in the legs. The most common yes–no questions addressed with an emergency medicine ultrasound of the lower extremity are those related to the presence of deep vein thrombosis (DVT).

ANATOMY

The anatomy of interest in the lower extremity vascular ultrasound involves the common femoral vein and the popliteal vein.
Common femoral vein
Saphenous vein
Common femoral artery
Popliteal vein
Popliteal artery

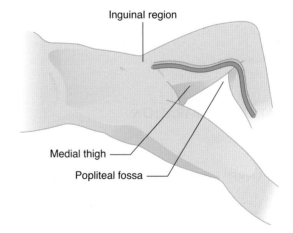

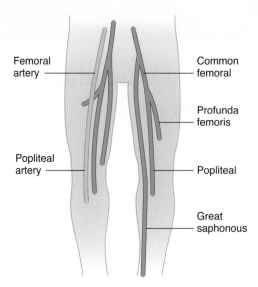

The lower extremity blood vessels enter at the inguinal crease and course around the medial thigh as they descend. Superiorly, the vein lies deep to the artery but this reverses behind the knee (popliteal fossa) with the artery deeper.

PATIENT POSITION

Common Femoral Vein

- Supine
- Leg in external rotation

Popliteal Vein

- Supine
- Leg flexed at knee
- Leg in external rotation,
    or
- Leg dangling over edge of examination table,
    or
- Prone position
- Leg flexed at knee

PATIENT PREPARATION

Not applicable

TRANSDUCER

5.0 to 7.5 MHz
Linear or wide footprint, curved ultrasound probe

LOWER EXTREMITY VASCULAR PATHOLOGY

- Inability to fully compress venous structures and decreased Doppler signal with calf augmentation (when compared to contralateral side) correspond to DVT

MANEUVERS

- Slightly bending the leg with external rotation allows easier access to the popliteal fossa
- Squeezing the lower extremity with one hand while imaging proximally with Doppler will detect augmented venous flow in a normal patient
- Arterial (pulsatile) and venous (phasic) Doppler wave forms are easily differentiated

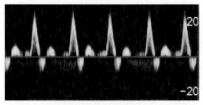
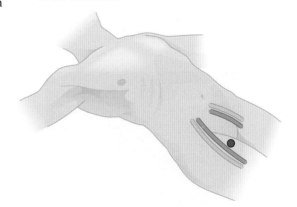

Arterial Tracing   Venous Tracing

LOWER EXTREMITY VASCULAR ESSENTIAL IMAGES

- Superior vasculature (transverse)
- Common femoral vein and artery
  - Start at level of great saphenous vein
  - Gray-scale image
  - Image with compression
- Lower vasculature (transverse)
- Popliteal vein and artery
  - Gray-scale image
  - Image with compression

Additional Images

- Common femoral vein and artery
  - Doppler
  - Doppler with augmentation
- Popliteal vein and artery
  - Doppler
  - Doppler with augmentation

Probe Placement

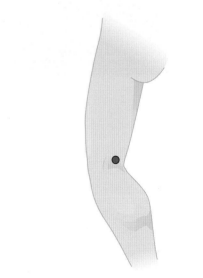

Each set of essential images (gray scale, compression) is repeated every 2 cm from the inguinal crease to the superior calf.

Tricks of the Trade

- Repeated external calf compressions can exhaust the venous reservoir and result in loss of flow pulse during augmentation.

- Deep veins are always paired but superficial vessels may be single.

- Keeping part of the hand holding the ultrasound probe in contact with the patient's skin will prevent inadvertent migration of the probe head during image acquisition.

- The primary criterion proven most useful in the diagnosis of DVT is gray-scale compression. Employing Doppler techniques such as augmentation only serves as an adjunct to the diagnosis, and should not be solely relied upon.

COMMON FEMORAL ARTERY AND VEIN

Landmarks

- Vein and artery outline
- Doppler signal (if needed)

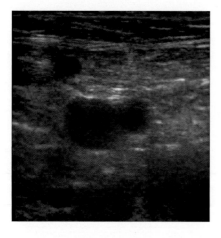
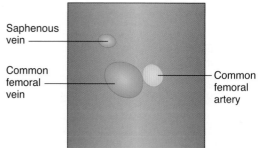

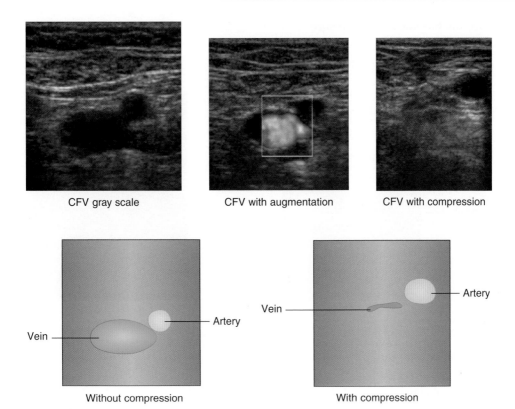

CFV gray scale   CFV with augmentation   CFV with compression

Vein ——   —— Artery

Without compression

Vein ——   —— Artery

With compression

Image Elements

- Artery contour
- Vein contour
- Vein internal architecture
- Compression of vessel
- Doppler signal (+/– augmentation)

Tricks of the Trade

- Using increased pressure when initially attempting to locate the common femoral vein may collapse it and limit visualization. Use gentle pressure when locating the veins as they compress easily.

- Older clots may adhere to the vessel wall, allowing flow proximally. Differentiation of chronic vs. acute clots requires advanced techniques beyond the scope of this textbook.

- Failure to use sufficient pressure to compress a vein may result in a false positive. Use enough pressure to cause slight dimpling of the skin. The artery is compressed when too much pressure is applied.

Too Much Initial Probe Pressure

Visualization of arteries and not veins
Same image as with intentional compression

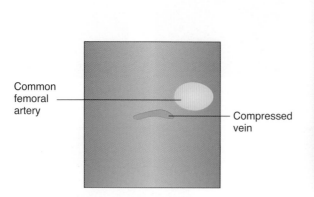

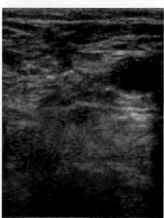

Popliteal vein and artery

Landmarks

- Vein and artery outline
- Doppler signal

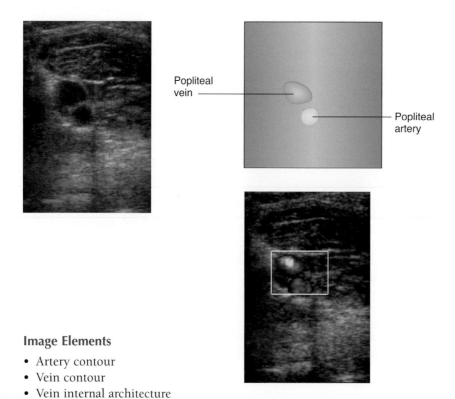

Image Elements

- Artery contour
- Vein contour
- Vein internal architecture
- Compression of vessel
- Doppler signal (+/– augmentation)

Tricks of the Trade

- It may be helpful to remember the rhyme: "The Vein Comes to the Top in the Pop", when deciding which vessel is venous in the popliteal fossa.

- In the popliteal fossa, the biceps femoris tendon may interfere with compression resulting in a false-positive ultrasound for intraluminal clot in the popliteal vein.

ULTRASOUND TECHNIQUE

Still Image Protocol

Common Femoral Vein and Artery: Short Axis

Approach – Transverse plane, anterior
     Transducer at inguinal crease
     Indicator toward patient's right side
     Probe perpendicular to skin
     Light pressure

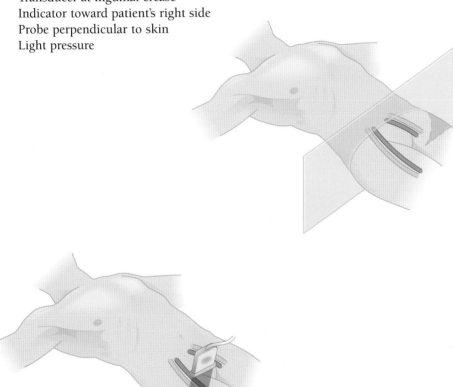

Images Required at Each Point of Common Femoral Vein

Paired images every 2 cm:
    Gray-scale static image
    Gray-scale image with compression of venous structures

Additional Images

Color flow Doppler image
Color flow Doppler image with venous augmentation
Compress calf or thigh while imaging
    (Note: The probe does not move during the two essential and two additional images.)

Popliteal Vein and Artery: Short Axis

Approach – Transverse plane, posterior
    Transducer at popliteal fossa
    Indicator toward patient's right side
    Probe perpendicular to skin
    Light pressure

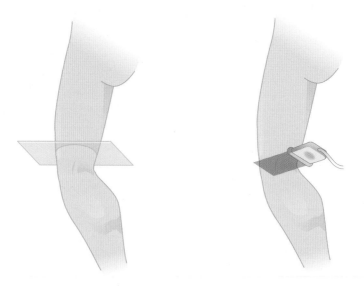

Images Required at Each Point of Popliteal Vein

Paired images every 2 cm:
    Gray-scale static image
    Gray-scale image with compression of venous structures

Optional Images

Color flow Doppler image
Color flow Doppler image with venous augmentation
     Compress calf while imaging
     (Note: The probe does not move during the two essential and two additional images.)

VIDEOTAPE PROTOCOL

Common Femoral Vein and Artery: Short Axis

Starting point – Transverse plane, anterior
     Transducer superior to inguinal crease
     Indicator toward patient's right side
     Probe perpendicular to skin
     Light pressure

Taping protocol

     Focus on silhouette of vein and artery
     Slide inferior toward knee
     Follow course of common femoral vein
     Compress vein in 2-cm increments
     Stop every 2 cm to repeat image sequence
     Continue until popliteal vein (see below)

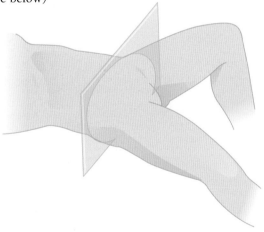

Popliteal Vein and Artery: Short Axis

Starting point – Transverse plane, anterior
    Transducer at popliteal fossa, as superior as possible
    Indicator toward patient's right side
    Probe perpendicular to skin
    Light pressure

Taping protocol
    Focus on silhouette of vein and artery
    Slide inferior toward ankle
    Follow course of popliteal vein
    Compress vein in 2-cm increments
    Stop every 2 cm to repeat image sequence
    Continue into calf until vein is not visualized

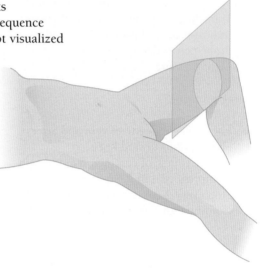

SMALL PARTS PROTOCOLS

Testicle Scanning Protocol

Paul Sierzenski

GOAL OF TESTICLE ULTRASOUND

Demonstrate abnormalities in the testicle and scrotum related to internal architecture, echogenicity, testicular contour, and blood flow. Additionally, fluid collections, cysts, and masses can be identified.

EMERGENCY ULTRASOUND APPROACH

Emergency medicine ultrasound of the testicle is focused on the clinical questions involving the scrotum and testicle. Patients with acute scrotal pain or testicular swelling are commonly seen in the emergency department. The most common yes–no question to be addressed for these patients is the presence or absence of testicular torsion.

A detailed understanding of all aspects of Doppler ultrasound is critical to the effective use of testicular ultrasound in emergency medicine. However, a complete discussion of Doppler ultrasound is beyond the scope of this book. Doppler imaging is a more complex application that many physicians may not feel comfortable attempting to master. As with all emergency ultrasound protocols a series of gray-scale images is critical prior to beginning any Doppler assessment.

There are two general ways that emergency ultrasound can be used in the workup of scrotal pain. Ultrasound can either "rule out" testicular torsion or diagnose an alternative, more common diagnosis such as epididymitis. In the first scenario ultrasound demonstrates equal arterial and venous flow within the symptomatic and asymptomatic testicles. In the second scenario ultrasound confirms the presence of findings that effectively exclude torsion, such as epididymitis/orchitis.

Many physicians who use testicular ultrasound use it in a limited capacity, specifically to include and support the diagnosis of epididymitis with or without orchitis, rather than the inclusion or exclusion of testicular torsion due to medical legal risks. In most cases immediate urological consultation should be considered unless it is clear that outpatient follow-up is appropriate.

ANATOMY

The anatomy of interest involves the testicle; its blood supply and the surrounding tissues.

- Testicular artery
- Epididymis
  - Head
  - Body
  - Tail
- Testicle
- Mediastinum testis
- Scrotal dermis

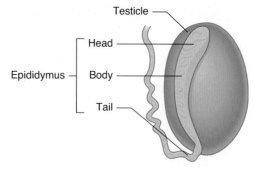

Posterior-lateral view

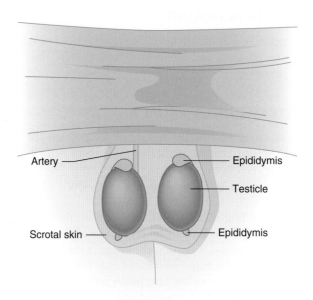

PATIENT POSITION

- Supine, with legs straight or in frog-leg position for comfort
- It is important to remember that patients presenting with testicular or scrotal pain may be reluctant to move

PATIENT PREPARATION

- Use several towels or drapes to isolate the scrotum, and have the patient's penis rest on the abdomen

TRANSDUCER

- 7.5 to 10 MHz linear probe

TESTICULAR PATHOLOGY

- Epididymitis results in relatively hypoechoic images of the epididymis
- Orchitis results in relatively hypoechoic images of the testicle
- Testicular torsion results in varied images depending on time to presentation

TESTIS ESSENTIAL IMAGES

- Right testicle
  - Testicle long axis
  - Testicle short axis
  - Epididymis
    - Head
    - Body
    - Tail
- Left testicle
  - Testicle long axis
  - Testicle short axis
  - Epididymis
    - Head
    - Body
    - Tail
- Bilateral testes – Transverse view

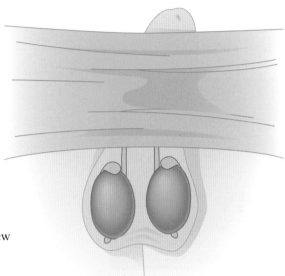

Compare testis color or power Doppler with sample box crossing regions of both testes simultaneously.

Tricks of the Trade
• Analgesia prior to imaging may improve image quality since any movement may result in flash artifacts for both color and spectral Doppler.
• A lower frequency probe (3.5–5.0 MHz) may be used in patients with a greatly enlarged scrotum but a higher frequency probe should be attempted first.
• Always image the asymptomatic testicle first.
• Stabilize the testicle with your non-scanning hand. Often doing this from below the testis with a towel is helpful as the testis can slide after gel is applied.
• Set the initial color/power Doppler gain, filter, PRF, and scale low enough so you can identify slow velocities within the testicle. Adjust these to eliminate overgained Doppler, flash artifacts, and phantom flow.

TESTICLE: LONG AXIS

Views of the long axis of the testes comprise superior and inferior views to include all aspects of the testicle and epididymis. Lateral or medial views of the long axis of the testicle are included to see the portion of the testes not images by a single long axis view.

TESTICLE: LONG AXIS, MIDDLE

Landmarks

- Testicular silhouette

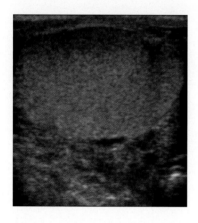
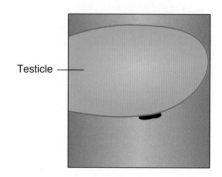

Image Elements

- Epididymis (head)
- Testicle
- Mediastinum testis
- Scrotal skin

Image Characteristics

- Testicle contour
- Testicle internal architecture
  - Homogenous (similar to liver)
- Testicle with color and spectral Doppler (both venous and arterial)

Doppler Images

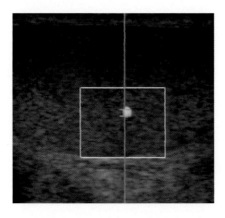

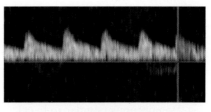

Arterial Tracing

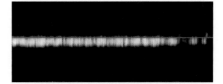

Venous Tracing

Tricks of the Trade

- All poor sagittal probe positions will result in the testis appearing smaller than actual size.

- Too lateral or too medial can result in identification of peripheral flow rather than central flow on color or spectral ultrasound. In chronic, intermittent, or late-presenting testicular torsion there can be increased peripheral testis flow but decreased central testis blood flow.

- Too superior or inferior transverse probe positions can result in identification of peripheral blood flow rather than central testis blood flow on color or spectral Doppler.

TESTICLE: LONG AXIS, SUPERIOR, OR EPIDIDYMIS HEAD, SAGITTAL

Landmarks

- Testicular silhouette
- Epididymis

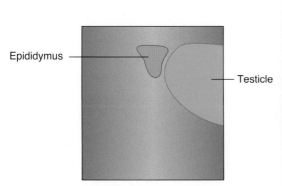

Epididymus —

 — Testicle

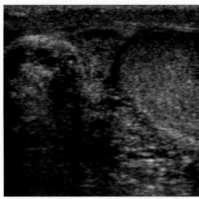

Image Elements

- Epididymis (head)
- Testicle
- Mediastinum testis (+/–)

Image Characteristics

- Testicle contour
- Testicle internal architecture
  - Homogenous (similar to liver)
- Epididymis internal architecture

TESTICLE: LONG AXIS, LATERAL OR MEDIAL

Landmarks

- Testicular silhouette

    (Note: Silhouette is similar to long axis but testicle appears smaller. The farther off axis the smaller the testicle will appear.)

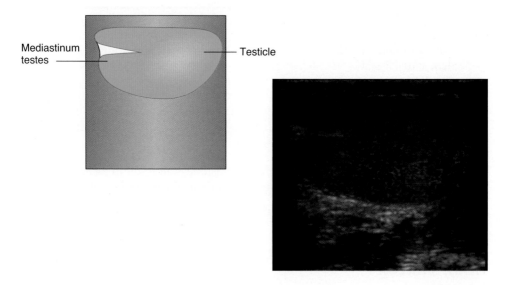

Mediastinum testes — — Testicle

Image Elements

- Testicle
- Mediastinum testis (+/–)

Image Characteristics

- Testicle contour
- Testicle internal architecture
  - Homogenous (similar to liver)
    - Epididymis internal architecture

TESTICLE: LONG AXIS, INFERIOR

Landmarks

- Testicular silhouette
- Epididymis

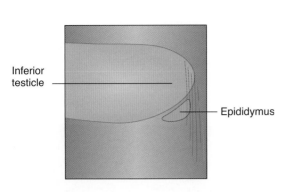 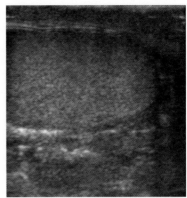

Image Elements
- Epididymis (tail)
- Testicle

Image Characteristics
- Testicle contour
- Testicle internal architecture
  - Homogenous (similar to liver)
- Epididymis internal architecture

Partial View Probe Positioning
The only partial view probe positionings of the testes demonstrate images where the probe extends off of the surface of the scrotum.

TESTICLE: SHORT AXIS, MIDDLE

Landmarks
- Testicular silhouette

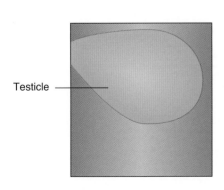 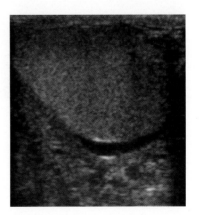

Image Elements
- Epididymis (head)
- Testicle
- Mediastinum testis

Image Characteristics

- Testicle contour
- Testicle internal architecture
  - Homogenous (similar to liver or thyroid)
- Testicle with color and spectral Doppler (both venous and arterial)

Doppler Images

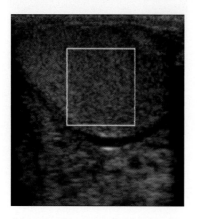

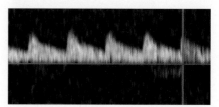

Arterial Tracing

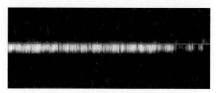

Venous Tracing

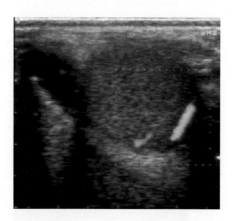

Tricks of the Trade

- Too lateral or too medial can result in identification of peripheral flow rather than central flow on color or spectral ultrasound. In chronic, intermittent, or late-presenting testicular torsion there can be increased peripheral testis flow but decreased central testis blood flow.

- Too superior or inferior transverse probe positions can result in identification of peripheral blood flow rather than central testis blood flow on color or spectral Doppler.

- Probe orientation for a transverse plane of testicle is variable as testicular lie may vary as a result of torsion, mass effect, or swelling.

TESTICLE: SHORT AXIS, SUPERIOR

Landmarks

- Testicular silhouette

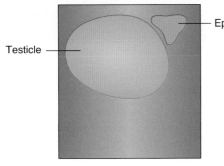

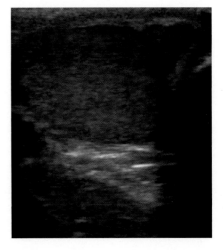

Image Elements

- Epididymis (+/−)
- Testicle
- Mediastinum testis (+/−)

Image Characteristics

- Testicle contour
- Testicle internal architecture
  - Homogenous (similar to liver or thyroid)

TESTICLE: SHORT AXIS, INFERIOR

Landmarks

- Testicular silhouette

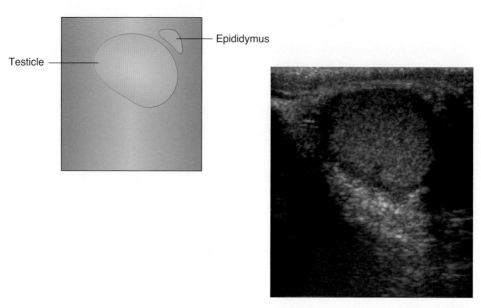

Image Elements

- Epididymis (+/−)
- Testicle
- Mediastinum testis (+/−)

Image Characteristics

- Testicle contour
- Testicle internal architecture
  - Homogenous (similar to liver)

Partial View Probe Positioning

The only partial view probe positionings of the testes demonstrate images where the probe extends off of the surface of the scrotum.

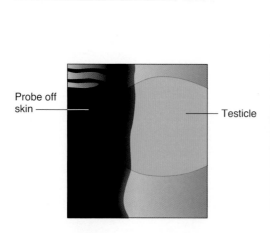

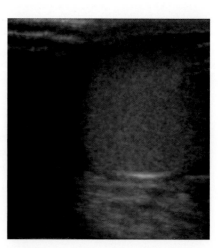

BILATERAL TESTICLE: SHORT AXIS

Landmarks

- Double testicle silhouette

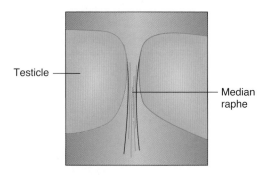

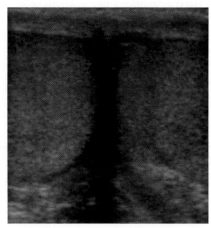

Image Elements

- Right testicle
- Left testicle
- Median raphe

Image Characteristics

- Testicle contour
- Testicle internal architecture
  - Homogenous (similar to liver)

Partial View Probe Positioning

Too Lateral

One testicle larger than the other

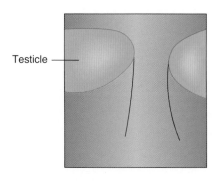

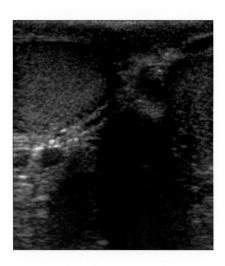

> *Tricks of the Trade*
>
> • A direct comparison of testicular tissue characteristics can be helpful in diagnosing testicular pathology.
>
> • Be careful of image orientation to accurately identify the appropriate testicle.
>
> • Clearly label right or left testicle to prevent confusion during later review.

ULTRASOUND TECHNIQUE

Still Image Protocol

Testicle: Long Axis, Sagittal

Approach – Sagittal plane, anterior
    Transducer on anterior surface of scrotum
    Indicator toward patient's head
    Midline of testicle
    Probe perpendicular to skin

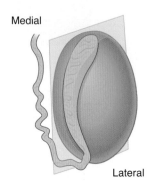

Medial

Lateral

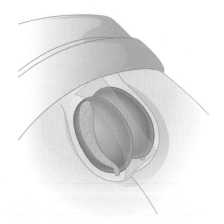
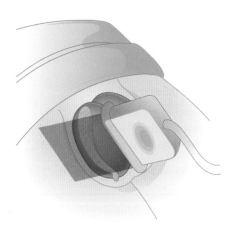

Include single or multiple images of medial and lateral testicle to completely image the testicle.

Testicle: Long Axis, Medial, Parasagittal

Approach – Sagittal plane, anterior
    Transducer on anterior surface of scrotum
    Indicator toward patient's head
    Medial portion of testicle
    Probe perpendicular to skin

Testicle: Long Axis, Lateral, Parasagittal

Approach – Sagittal plane, anterior
    Transducer on anterior surface of scrotum
    Indicator toward patient's head
    Lateral portion of testicle
    Probe perpendicular to skin

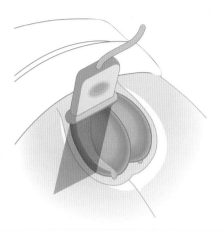

Testicle: Short Axis, Superior

Approach – Transverse plane, anterior
    Transducer on anterior surface of scrotum
    Indicator toward patient's right
    Superior testicle
    Probe perpendicular to skin

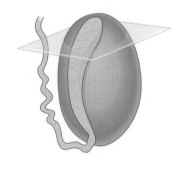

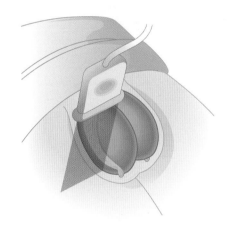

Testicle: Short Axis, Middle

Approach – Transverse plane, anterior
    Transducer on anterior surface of scrotum
    Indicator toward patient's right
    Middle of testicle
    Probe perpendicular to skin

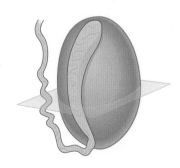

Testicle: Short Axis, Inferior

Approach – Transverse plane, anterior
    Transducer on anterior surface of scrotum
    Indicator toward patient's right
    Inferior testicle
    Probe perpendicular to skin

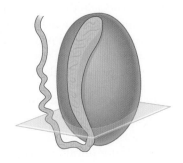

Bilateral Testicle: Short Axis

Approach – Transverse plane, anterior
    Transducer on anterior surface of scrotum
    Probe over middle of scrotum
    Indicator toward patient's right
    Probe perpendicular to skin

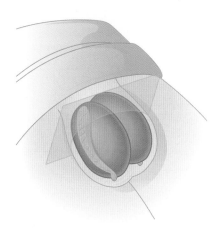 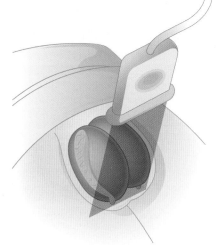

Single Testicle: Doppler Images

Long or short axis
Same approach as with gray scale
Find intratesticular tissue with representative blood flow
Color or power Doppler imaging
Spectral imaging

Bilateral Testicle: Doppler Images

Short axis
Same approach as with gray scale
Find intratesticular tissue with representative blood flow
Color or power Doppler imaging
Spectral imaging

Testicle: Long Axis, Coronal or Sagittal

Approach – Coronal (or sagittal) plane, inferior

> Transducer on inferior surface of scrotum
>
> Indicator toward patient's right (or ceiling)
>
> Probe perpendicular to skin, parallel to stretcher
>
> (Note: This view may aid in Doppler signal identification as blood flow to the testis begins superior to inferior along the course of the testicular and deferential arteries.)

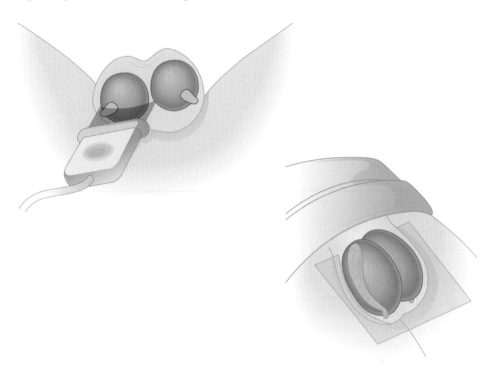

VIDEOTAPE PROTOCOL

Testicle: Long Axis

Starting point – Sagittal plane, anterior

> Transducer on anterior surface of scrotum
>
> Indicator toward patient's head
>
> Midline of testicle
>
> Probe perpendicular to skin

Taping protocol

> Focus on silhouette of testicle
>
> Sweep medial to lateral
>
> Scan entire width of testicle
>
> Include entire length of testicle
>
> Hold long axis view of testicle
>
> Color Doppler and spectral Doppler images

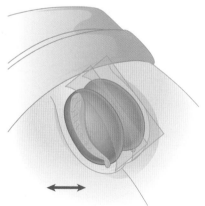

Testicle: Short Axis

Starting point – Transverse plane, anterior
 Transducer on anterior surface of scrotum
 Indicator toward patient's right side
 Midline of testicle
 Probe perpendicular to skin

Taping protocol
 Focus on silhouette of testicle
 Sweep superior to inferior
 Scan entire length of testicle
 Include entire width of testicle
 Hold midline short axis view of testicle
 Color Doppler and spectral Doppler images

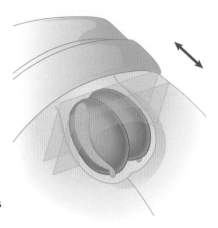

Bilateral Testes: Short Axis

Starting point – Transverse plane, anterior
 Transducer on anterior surface of scrotum
 Indicator toward patient's right side
 Midline of scrotum
 Probe perpendicular to skin

Taping protocol
 Focus on equal silhouette of both testicles
 Sweep superior to inferior
 Scan entire length of testicle
 Hold midline short axis view of testicle
 Color Doppler and spectral Doppler image

Ocular Scanning Protocol

Paul Sierzenski

GOAL OF OCULAR ULTRASOUND

Demonstrate abnormalities of the eye related to abnormal ocular architecture.

EMERGENCY ULTRASOUND APPROACH

Emergency medicine ultrasound of the eye is focused on the clinical questions involving the eye. Patients with acute eye pain or visual complaints often will present to the emergency department for evaluation. The most common yes–no question to be addressed for these patients is that of retinal detachment. Other pathologic conditions of the eye such as intraocular foreign body, vitreous hemorrhage, increased optic nerve sheath diameter (associated with increased intracranial pressure), retrobulbar hematoma, and lens dislocation can be diagnosed with ultrasound. If an open globe rupture is suspected, ocular ultrasound is contraindicated.

ANATOMY

- Anterior chamber
- Lens
- Posterior chamber
- Retina
- Optic nerve sheath
- Retrobulbar space

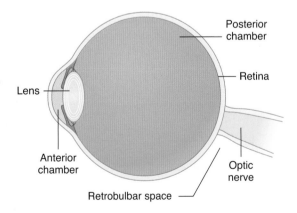

PATIENT POSITION

- Supine
- Semi-erect with the head of the bed at about 30 degrees

PATIENT PREPARATION

- Scan through a closed eye
- Use ample gel directly on the closed lid
- Little or no direct pressure on the globe itself

TRANSDUCER

- High frequency linear – 7.5 to 10 MHz or potentially higher (12–15 MHz)
- Lowest power settings (increased gain) that allow visualization (if adjustable)

ULTRASOUND IMAGES

Ocular Essential Images

- Eye (right and left)
  - Longitudinal
  - Transverse
- Retrobulbar space
- Optic nerve sheath

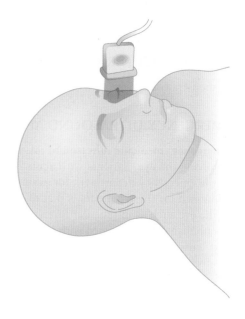

EYE: TRANSVERSE AXIS

Landmarks

- Ocular silhouette

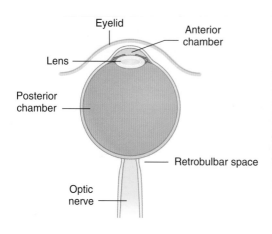

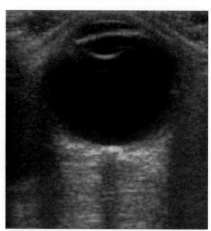

Image Elements

- Lens
- Anterior chamber
- Posterior chamber
- Retrobulbar space
- Optic nerve sheath

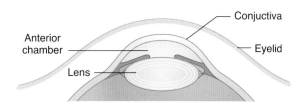

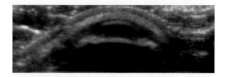

Tricks of the Trade

- Image the asymptomatic eye first for comparison.

- Use ample gel. The eye sits somewhat recessed below the surrounding orbit and its ridge.

- Stabilize your hand over the bridge of the nose and the forehead.

- Consider keeping the probe stationary while having the patient move the eye under a closed lid to fully evaluate the orbit.

- Cooling the ultrasound gel will increase its viscosity and help to keep it in the orbit.

- Common artifacts cause poor imaging of the "sides" of the eye and false echoes within the posterior chamber.

Partial View Probe Positioning

Note: Most partial views of the eye show some but not all of the elements listed above. With most atypical probe placements there will be no visualization of the eye.

EYE: LONGITUDINAL AXIS

Note: With normal anatomy, images in longitudinal axis will appear identical to images in transverse axis.

Landmarks

• Ocular silhouette

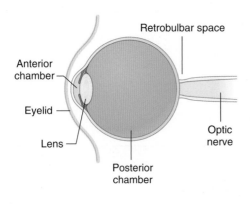
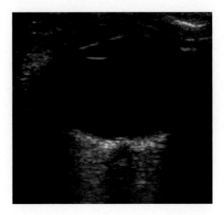

Image Elements

• Lens
• Anterior chamber
• Posterior chamber
• Retrobulbar space
• Optic nerve sheath

Partial View Probe Positioning

Note: Most partial views of the eye show some but not all of the elements listed above. With most atypical probe placements there will be no visualization of the eye.

ULTRASOUND TECHNIQUE

Still Image Protocol

Eye: Longitudinal Axis, Midline

Approach – Sagittal, anterior
Transducer centered over closed eyelid
Indicator toward patient's forehead
Probe perpendicular to face (initially)
Orient probe through anterior chamber and optic nerve sheath

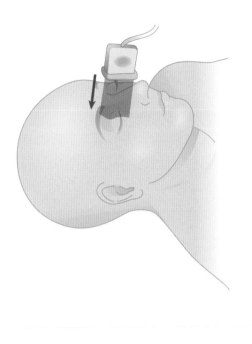

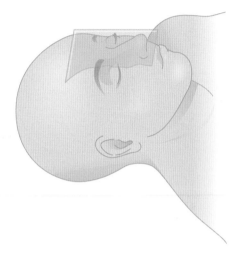

Eye: Longitudinal Axis, Lateral

Approach – Sagittal, anterior
    Transducer lateral side of orbit
    Indicator toward patient's forehead
    Probe perpendicular to face (initially)
    Orient probe parallel to midline view

Eye: Longitudinal Axis, Medial

Approach – Sagittal, anterior
    Transducer nasal side of orbit
    Indicator toward patient's forehead
    Probe perpendicular to face (initially)
    Orient probe parallel to midline view

Lens: Longitudinal Axis

Approach – Sagittal, anterior
    Transducer centered over closed eyelid
    Indicator toward patient's forehead
    Probe perpendicular to face
    Center lens in image

Eye: Transverse Axis, Midline

Approach – Transverse, anterior
    Transducer centered over closed eyelid
    Indicator toward patient's right side
    Probe perpendicular to face
    Orient probe through anterior chamber and optic nerve sheath

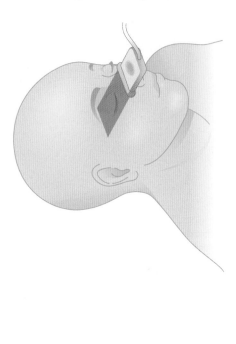

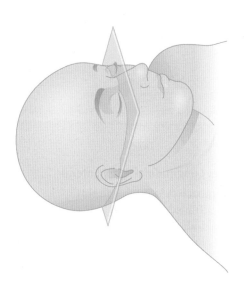

Eye: Transverse Axis, Superior

Approach – Transverse, anterior
    Transducer superior orbit
    Indicator toward patient's right side
    Probe perpendicular to face
    Orient probe parallel to midline view

Eye: Transverse Axis, Inferior

Approach – Transverse, anterior
    Transducer inferior orbit
    Indicator toward patient's right side
    Probe perpendicular to face
    Orient probe parallel to midline view

Lens: Transverse Axis

Approach – Transverse, anterior
    Transducer centered over orbit
    Indicator toward patient's right side
    Probe perpendicular to face
    Center lens in image

VIDEOTAPE PROTOCOL

Eye: Longitudinal Axis

Starting point – Sagittal plane, anterior
Transducer centered over orbit
Indicator toward patient's forehead
Probe perpendicular to face
Orient probe through anterior chamber and optic nerve sheath

Taping protocol
Center eye (anterior and posterior chamber) in image
Sweep medial to lateral and back
Sweep entire width of eye
Include images of optic nerve sheath
Include detailed images of lens and anterior chamber

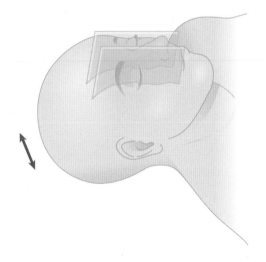

Eye: Transverse Axis

Starting point – Transverse plane, anterior
    Transducer centered over orbit
    Indicator toward patient's right side
    Probe perpendicular to face
    Orient probe through anterior chamber and optic nerve sheath

Taping protocol
    Center eye (anterior and posterior chamber) in image
    Sweep superior to inferior and back
    Sweep entire length of eye
    Include images of optic nerve sheath
    Include detailed images of lens and anterior chamber

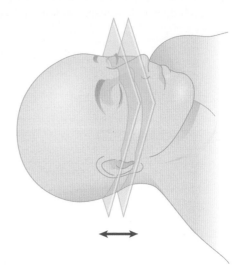

NON-PROTOCOL DRIVEN ULTRASOUND

GOAL OF NON-PROTOCOL DRIVEN ULTRASOUND

This chapter will focus on ultrasounds that are not protocol driven. Non-protocol driven ultrasound focuses on clinical decisions prior to an invasive procedure or ultrasound imaging for guidance of an invasive procedure. Because these ultrasounds can vary widely in terms of probe location, pathology, and anatomy, this chapter is procedure driven rather than protocol driven. As with all applications of bedside ultrasound, documentation of the images using either still or video imagery is a necessary component of this practice.

NON-PROTOCOL ULTRASOUND AND PROCEDURE

Musculoskeletal Ultrasound

- Soft tissue ultrasound (ultrasound guided)
  Question – Abscess vs. cellulitis
  Procedure – Incision and drainage
- Soft tissue ultrasound (ultrasound guided)
  Question – Location of foreign body
  Procedure – Removal of foreign body
- Chest and chest wall imaging (ultrasound prior to procedure)
  Question – Detection of pneumothorax
  Procedure – Chest tube insertion
- Spinal ultrasound
  Question – Location of spinous processes
  Procedure – Lumbar puncture

Ultrasound Guided Central Line Placement

- Vascular ultrasound (ultrasound guided)
  Question – Location of internal jugular vein
  Procedure – Central venous catheterization
- Vascular ultrasound (ultrasound guided)
  Question – Location of common femoral vein
  Procedure – Central venous catheterization

Ultrasound Guided Fluid Drainage

- Chest and chest wall imaging (ultrasound guided)
  Question – Detection of pleural fluid
  Procedure – Thoracentesis
  Question – Detection of pericardial fluid
  Procedure – Pericardiocentesis
- Abdominal imaging (ultrasound guided procedure)
  Question – Detection of peritoneal fluid
  Procedure – Paracentesis

Skin and Soft Tissue Ultrasound

13

J. Christian Fox and Romolo Gaspari

GOAL OF SOFT TISSUE ULTRASOUND

Demonstrate abnormal structures in skin or superficial connective tissue or muscle.

ANATOMY

Anatomy of interest depends on the location of the ultrasound.
- Skin
- Muscle
- Tendon
- Bony structures
- Vessels

    Use known structures such as muscle, bone, and vessels as landmarks to reference the mass or object in question. These landmarks will vary depending on their location. For example, neck masses will have muscle, vascular, and thyroid tissue surrounding them, whereas abdominal wall masses will tend to have more fat and muscle surrounding them. Masses located in the extremities will typically have bony shadows, vessels, and muscle tissue as landmarks.

CLINICAL QUESTION

- Cystic vs. solid mass
- Abscess vs. cellulitis
- Location of foreign body

    The answer to this question has clinical implications for possible future outpatient workup or immediate bedside interventions.

PATIENT POSITION

- Varies depending on area being imaged

PATIENT PREPARATION

- Remove distal jewelry
- Clean skin of debris and particulate matter
- Disinfect skin

TRANSDUCER

- High frequency linear probe

ULTRASOUND APPEARANCE OF SKIN AND SOFT TISSUE PATHOLOGY

- Solid (echogenic mass)
- Cystic structure (anechoic round cyst with posterior enhancement)
- Hematoma (variable depending on time from onset)
- Foreign body (appearance depends on foreign body material and presence or absence of gas or surrounding fluid)
- Abscess (hypoechoic with irregular borders)
- Cellulitis (hyperechoic "islands" surrounded by small anechoic "lakes")

ULTRASOUND IMAGES

- Long axis of area being imaged
- Short axis of area being imaged

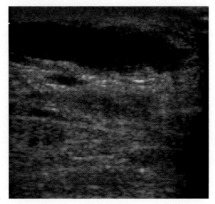

Long Axis

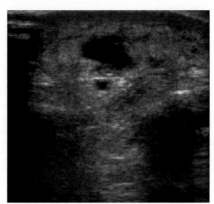

Short Axis

ULTRASOUND TECHNIQUE: GENERAL

- Position area of interest in center of monitor
  - Line center of probe over area of interest
- Rotate probe 90 degrees counterclockwise and re-image
- Identify surrounding items of interest
  (Example: Subcutaneous structure in groin—identify femoral artery, vein)

Abscess vs. Cellulitis

Bedside ultrasound answers the clinical question of whether or not an erythematous region of the skin also harbors a surgically drainable abscess beneath.

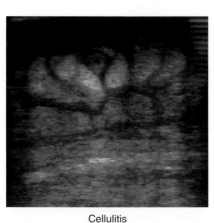

Cellulitis

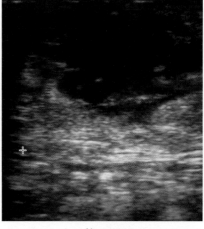

Abscess

Probe Selection

- 5 to 7.5 MHz or higher
- Linear
- Highest resolution setting

Ultrasound Technique: Abscess

- Position probe over center of swelling or redness
- Locate boundaries of fluid collection
- Identify surrounding structures for location

(Example: Abscess extends to bony surface of 3rd metacarpal)

- Identify structures that may complicate incision and drainage (I & D)

(Example: Abscess of wrist near radial artery)

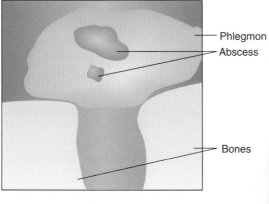

Phlegmon
Abscess

Bones

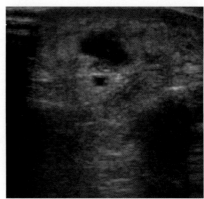

Procedure Technique

Needle aspiration (static guidance)
- Identify boundaries of abscess and corresponding surface landmarks
- Mark or identify where needle will penetrate skin and angle of introduction of needle
- Disinfect skin prior to introduction of needle
- Introduce needle into skin
- Aspirate while advancing needle into abscess
- Repeat if needed

Needle aspiration (dynamic guidance)
- Disinfect skin prior to ultrasound
- Identify largest area of fluid collection (probe in sterile cover)
- Place area of fluid collection in center of screen
- Introduce needle next to probe at center angling toward abscess
- Aspirate as needle is advanced
- Image needle as it penetrates abscess

Incision and drainage (static guidance)
- Identify boundaries of abscess and corresponding surface landmarks
- Mark or identify where scalpel will cut skin (most superficial fluid collection or largest fluid collection)
- Disinfect skin prior to incision
- Incision of skin with blunt dissection of septations or loculations
- Express with pressure around incision
- Repeat as needed
- Leave incision open and pack with sterile packing material

Incision and drainage (dynamic guidance)
- Identify boundaries of abscess and corresponding surface landmarks
- Mark or identify where scalpel will cut skin (most superficial fluid collection or largest fluid collection)
- Disinfect skin prior to incision
- Introduce scalpel directly under center of probe
- Ultrasound probe is removed once purulent material is encountered.

Tricks of the Trade

- Cellulitis with localized edema will have low-level echoes in the "anechoic" space and can look like an abscess.

- Gas-forming abscesses will cause comet tail artifacts that can blur the edges of the abscess.

- Be conscious of identifying foreign bodies within the body of an abscess.

- Re-image area of abscess following I & D or needle aspiration to monitor drainage.

- Compression of an abscess often results in streaming or swirling of pus.

- For deeper abscesses it may be necessary to use the lower range of frequencies or even a curved probe set to its higher frequency setting.

- To identify point of incision during I & D locate probe over most superficial fluid collection, not largest fluid collection.

Image Elements
- Body of abscess
- Boundaries of abscess
- Surrounding landmarks
- Needle penetration (for ultrasound guided aspiration)

Still Image Protocol
Use known structures such as muscle, bone, and vessels as landmarks to reference the abscess in question. These landmarks will vary depending on their location.

Preprocedure Imaging
Identify longest length of abscess
Identify surrounding anatomy
Demonstrate abscess in two perpendicular planes

Periprocedure Imaging
Image needle penetrating abscess (in one plane)

Postprocedure Imaging
Image drained abscess cavity
Identify any remaining fluid collections

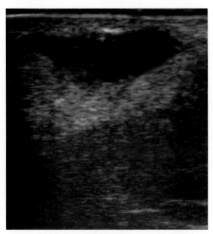

Pre-needle

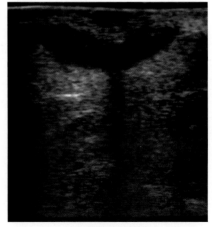

During Needle

Videotape Protocol

Initial Image of Abscess

Identify longest length of abscess
Fan side to side
Image entire abscess
Identify surrounding anatomy
Rotate 90 degrees counterclockwise
Fan from top to bottom
Identify surrounding structures

Procedure Documentation (Real-Time Guidance of Needle Aspiration Only)

Find largest pocket of fluid
Image needle as it penetrates abscess
Postprocedure imaging
Image drained abscess cavity
Identify any remaining fluid collections

FOREIGN BODY REMOVAL

Localization and removal of a foreign body can be a time-consuming task often with fruitless results. Use of bedside ultrasound helps to pinpoint and retrieve the object in a timely fashion.

Probe Selection

- High frequency linear probe (at highest frequency)

Ultrasound Technique: Foreign Body Localization

- Position probe over area of interest (i.e., entrance wound)
- Slowly scan area of maximal interest
- Be willing to scan wider area if foreign body is not visualized initially
- Foreign bodies appear as highly echogenic structures that reflect sound in a way that can cause reverberation artifacts or shadows.
- Identify surrounding structures for localizing foreign body

Procedure Technique: Foreign Body Removal

- Locate foreign body
- Center foreign body on screen
- Introduce a needle along face of probe towards foreign body
- When needle contacts foreign body, remove ultrasound
- Incise down length of needle
- Remove foreign body

Tricks of the Trade

- Most foreign bodies are located very close to the skin surface and adequate visualization may require a standoff structure (e.g., a 250-cc bag of normal saline).

- Most foreign bodies are not easily visualized on ultrasound regardless of if they are seen on x-ray.

- "Creeping" the probe along the skin may identify weak artifact signals from smaller foreign bodies that are not apparent when moving the probe quickly.

- Foreign bodies within an abscess may be silhouetted and easier to identify.

- Set a time frame when attempting to localize a foreign body and quit when time is up to prevent spending too much time on the procedure.

Image Elements

- Foreign body
- Artifact from foreign body
- Surrounding landmarks

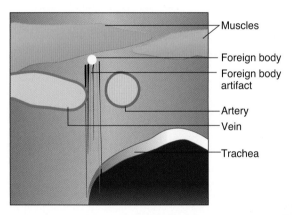

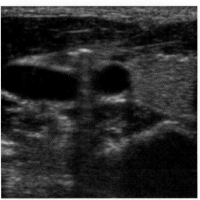

Still Image Protocol

Use known structures such as muscle, bone, and vessels as landmarks to reference the location of the foreign body. These landmarks will vary depending on the location of the foreign body.

- Identify foreign body or artifact of foreign body
- Identify surrounding landmarks

Videotape Protocol

Video documentation of ultrasound uses the same landmarks and positioning as stills, but video allows for a dynamic documentation of the foreign body removal.

Chest Wall Ultrasound for Pneumothorax

14

Romolo Gaspari and J. Christian Fox

GOAL OF CHEST WALL ULTRASOUND

Identification of pneumothorax.

RATIONALE FOR CHEST WALL ULTRASOUND

Using ultrasound allows you to identify the chest wall and pleural lining of the lung. A pneumothorax may result in requiring the placement of a chest tube to reinflate the lung.

ANATOMY

- Ribs
- Lung
- Pleura (lining of lung)
- Intercostal muscle

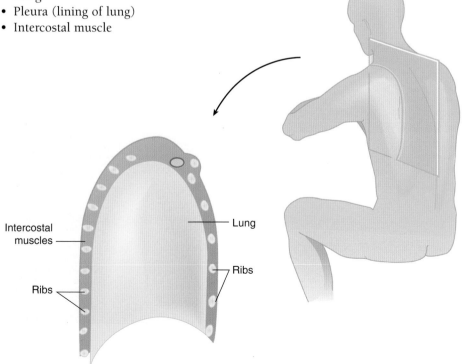

Intercostal muscles

Lung

Ribs

Ribs

PATIENT POSITION

- Supine

PATIENT PREPARATION

- None

TRANSDUCER

- High-frequency linear probe

ULTRASOUND IMAGE ELEMENTS

- Ribs
- Lung edge (pleura)
- Chest wall–lung interface

ULTRASOUND APPEARANCE OF PNEUMOTHORAX

- During normal respiration the lung and chest wall "slide" past one another
- Comet tail artifact (small white linear streaks) radiate away from the probe surface and migrate back and forth during respiration
- Absence of normal findings indicate pneumothorax

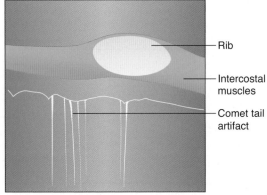

Rib

Intercostal muscles

Comet tail artifact

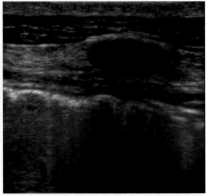

ULTRASOUND TECHNIQUE

- Position probe on anterior chest wall
- Over 2nd–3rd or 3rd–4th rib space
- Mid-clavicular line, *or*, just lateral to sternum
- Indicator to patient's head
- Hold probe between superior and inferior rib
- Hold probe stationary through multiple respiratory cycles

Tricks of the Trade

- Using M-mode provides alternative proof of pneumothorax. Place M-mode cursor between the rib shadows and observe a tracing consistent with lung sliding. A pneumothorax produces a continuous straight line along the M-mode tracing.

- It is difficult to demonstrate a pneumothorax using still images alone.

- Color power Doppler imaging of the chest wall–lung interface should show a signal flare in normal lung.

Still Image Protocol

Approach – Sagittal plane, anterior
    Transducer on anterior chest
    Mid-clavicular line, *or*, just lateral to sternum
    Indicator toward head
    Probe perpendicular to skin
    Hold probe still during respiratory cycle

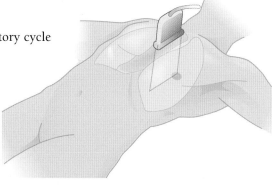

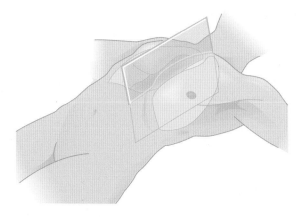

Videotape Protocol

Video documentation of ultrasound uses the same landmarks and positioning as stills, but video allows for a dynamic documentation of the sliding lung. There is no movement of probe during recording of ultrasound.

Ultrasound Guided Lumbar Puncture

15

J. Christian Fox and Romolo Gaspari

GOAL OF ULTRASOUND GUIDED LUMBAR PUNCTURE

Facilitate placement of spinal needle during lumbar puncture.

RATIONALE FOR ULTRASOUND GUIDED LUMBAR PUNCTURE

Using ultrasound allows you to identify landmarks that are not palpable due to body habitus. In cases where anatomic landmarks are easily palpable, ultrasound guidance is not needed.

ANATOMY

- Spinous process
- Interspinal disk space
- Connective tissue

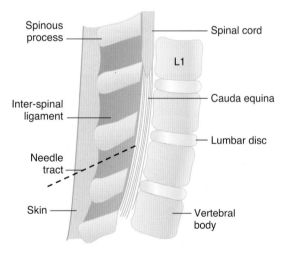

The bony landmarks appear as hyperechoic linear structures that completely reflect the sound, resulting in very distinct shadowing. When the probe is between two vertebrae, the intense reflection is no longer present and tissue can be visualized. It is between the bony landmarks that the needle needs to be directed to successfully obtain spinal fluid.

PATIENT POSITION

- Sitting up, leaning forward, *or*
- Lateral decubitus
- Lumbar flexion
- Line up hips and shoulders to keep spine strait

PATIENT PREPARATION

- Clean and disinfect skin

TRANSDUCER

- High frequency linear probe (5–10 MHz)

ULTRASOUND IMAGE ELEMENTS

- Spinous process
- Intervertebral disk space

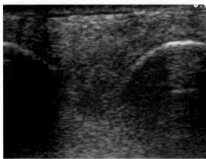 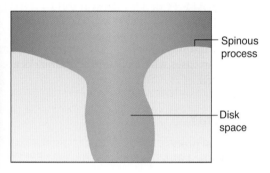

Spinous process

Disk space

Long Axis Spinous Process

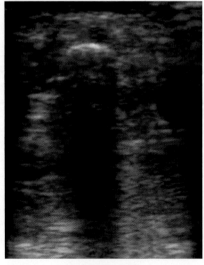 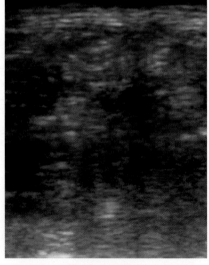

Transverse View
at Spinous Process

Transverse View
between Spinous Process

ULTRASOUND TECHNIQUE

- Position probe on midline of back
- Indicator orientation is toward the head (long axis) (preferred), *or*
- Indicator towards right side
- Locate intervertebral space

Procedure Technique

Still guidance
- Place patient in proper position
- Identify disk space
- Mark location for needle insertion
- Remove probe and disinfect skin
- Anesthetize skin surface
- Insert needle at predetermined spot on back

Dynamic guidance
- Disinfect skin surface
- Place probe in sterile cover
- Place patient in proper position
- Identify disk space
- Remove probe
- Anesthetize skin surface over disk space
- Re-image disk space
- Move probe slightly to one side
- Insert needle next to probe head at exact center of probe, angled slightly cephalad in relation to spine axis
- Remove probe and continue lumbar puncture

Alternative approach
- Paramedian approach
- Place ultrasound probe on patient's back
- Indicator towards head
- 2–4 cm lateral to midline
- Angle towards midline
- Identify disk space
- Mark spot for needle insertion site
- Remove probe from skin surface
- Sterilize skin surface
- Insert needle

Tricks of the Trade

- If anatomic landmarks are palpable then ultrasound guidance is not needed.

- Spinous processes are regularly repeating structures. Locating multiple superior spinal shadows give secondary indications where lower landmarks are located.

- Flexing the lumbar spine as much as possible enlarges the disk space for introduction of the needle.

- With linear probes with a large footprint the length probe will span two vertebral transverse processes when placed in the sagittal plane. The left side of the monitor will show the superior vertebral shadow and the right side will show the inferior vertebral shadow. The needle should be placed between the two shadows.

- Dynamic guidance during a lumbar puncture increases procedural complexity. Static guidance is usually adequate.

Still Image Protocol

Approach – Posterior, longitudinal
     Transducer at midline of back
     Indicator toward head
     Probe perpendicular to skin
     Locate probe over L3 or L4 disk space
     Image disk space

Videotape Protocol

Video documentation of ultrasound uses the same landmarks and positioning as stills, but video allows for a dynamic documentation locating the disk space or introducing the needle into the disk space. There is no movement of probe during procedure.

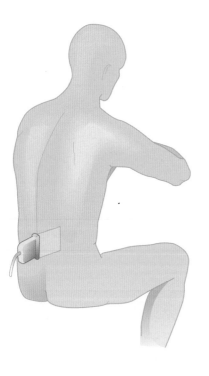
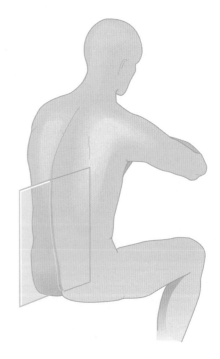

Vascular Procedure Ultrasound

J. Christian Fox and Romolo Gaspari

VASCULAR ULTRASOUND

Central Venous Cannulation

Goal of Ultrasound for Central Venous Cannulation

Facilitate placement of a venous catheter into a central vein.

Rationale for Ultrasound Guided Central Line Placement

- Ultrasound imaging allows you to align the probe, the vein, and the needle tip
- Visualization under real-time guidance reduces complications resulting from multiple attempts

One vs. Two Operator Technique

One operator technique
- Probe in one hand
- Introducer needle in other

Two operator technique
- One person holds probe
- The other person advances needle

ULTRASOUND GUIDED INTERNAL JUGULAR VEIN CANNULATION

Anatomy

Use known structures such as muscle and vessels as landmarks
- Internal jugular vein
- Subclavian vein
- Carotid artery
- Trachea
- Neck muscles

Patient Position

- Supine
- Trendelenburg
- Head turned to left (for right internal jugular)
- Head turned to right (for left internal jugular)

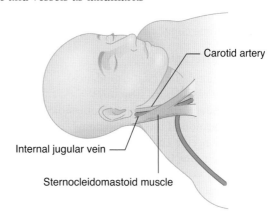

Carotid artery

Internal jugular vein

Sternocleidomastoid muscle

Patient Preparation

- Clean and disinfect skin

Transducer

- High frequency linear probe

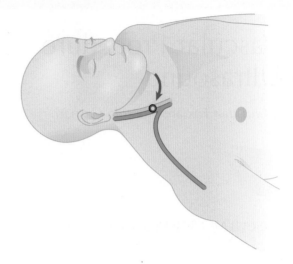

Ultrasound Image Elements

- Internal jugular vein
- Carotid artery
- Sternocleidomastoid muscle
- Trachea
- Needle tip, *or*, ring down artifact

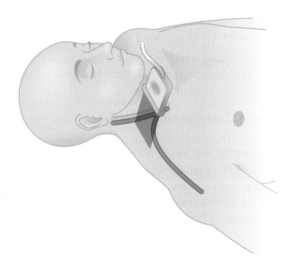

Ultrasound Technique

- Position probe on right lateral neck (right internal jugular)
- Indicator to patient's right
- Center internal jugular vein on screen
- Hold probe completely still during needle advancement

Procedure Technique

Venous cannulation (static guidance)
- Identify vasculature structures
- Avoid puncturing sternocleidomastoid muscle
- Note location of internal anatomy in relation to external anatomy
- Identify needle entry point on skin
- Remove probe from skin
- Disinfect skin prior to introducing needle
- Insert central line at predetermined point using Seldinger technique

Venous cannulation (dynamic guidance)
- Identify vascular structures
- Avoid puncturing sternocleidomastoid muscle
- Identify needle entry point
  - Hold needle at center of ultrasound probe, same distance from probe as vein is deep to probe (see figure)
- Introduce needle at 45-degree angle
- Image needle as it enters vein
  - Wall distends inward as needle pushes in
  - Wall snaps back outward as needle punctures wall

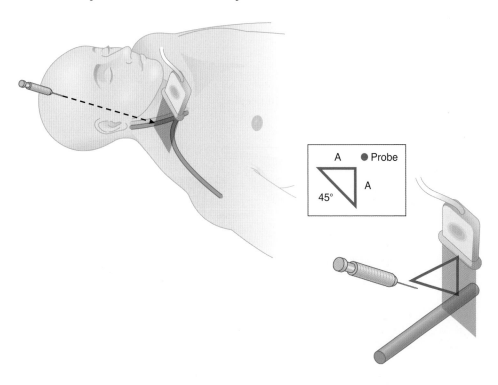

Tricks of the Trade

- Having the patient perform a Valsalva maneuver distends the vein and increases the chances of a successful line placement.

- The walls of the vein may tent inward when the needle approaches the vein. Extreme tenting (i.e., low vascular volume) may result in complete penetration of the anterior and posterior vein wall.

- Redirecting the needle once inside the patient during a difficult line placement will most likely result in no ultrasound guidance of the procedure. If the first pass is unsuccessful then remove needle from patient and start again from the beginning.

- The anatomy of the neck is mobile. If the patient moves (i.e., turns the head) after the static ultrasound but prior to inserting the needle, then the patient must be re-imaged prior to attempting line placement.

- Small rapid in-line movements of the needle (i.e., jiggling) during line placement will locate the needle tip on the screen by transmitting these movements to surrounding tissue.

- Jugular veins become noncompressible when a clot is contained within their lumen. Always confirm patency of the jugular vein by compressing it prior to cannulation attempt. If not compressible, consider using the contralateral side.

Still Image Protocol

Approach – Transverse plane, anterior
     Transducer at right lateral neck
     Indicator toward right side
     Probe perpendicular to skin
     Image vein prior to introduction of needle
     Image vein during introduction of needle

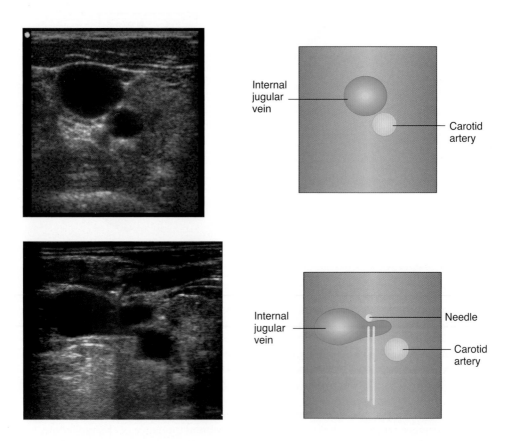

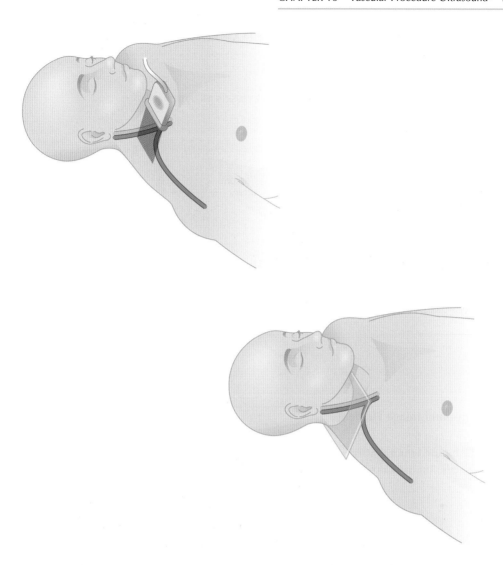

Videotape Protocol

Video documentation of ultrasound uses the same landmarks and positioning as stills, but video allows for a dynamic documentation of the introduction of the needle into the vein. There is no movement of probe during procedure.

ULTRASOUND GUIDED COMMON FEMORAL VEIN CANNULATION

Anatomy

Use known structures such as muscles and vessels as landmarks
- Common femoral vein
- Common femoral artery
- Great saphenous vein

Patient Position

- Supine
- Reverse Trendelenburg

Patient Preparation

- Clean and disinfect skin

Transducer

- High-frequency linear probe

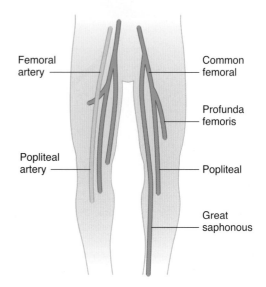

Ultrasound Image Elements

- Common femoral vein
- Common femoral artery
- Needle tip, ring down artifact

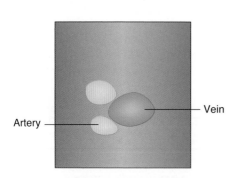

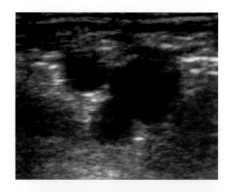

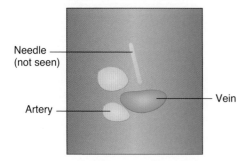

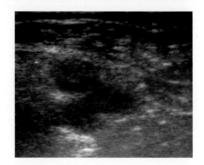

Ultrasound Technique

- Position probe on right or left thigh at inguinal ligament
- Indicator to patient's right
- Center common femoral vein on screen
- Hold probe completely still during needle advancement

Procedure Technique

Venous cannulation (static guidance)
- Identify vasculature structures
- Note location of internal anatomy in relation to external anatomy
- Identify needle entry point on skin
- Disinfect skin prior to introducing needle
- Remove probe from skin surface
- Anesthetize skin surface
- Insert central line at predetermined point using Seldinger technique

Venous Cannulation (Dynamic Guidance)

- Identify vascular structures
- Identify needle entry point
  - Hold needle at center of ultrasound probe, same distance from probe as vein is deep to probe (see figure below)
- Anesthetize skin surface
- Introduce needle at 45-degree angle
- Image needle as it enters vein
  - Wall distends inward as needle pushes in
  - Wall snaps back outward as needle punctures wall
- Complete line placement using Seldinger technique

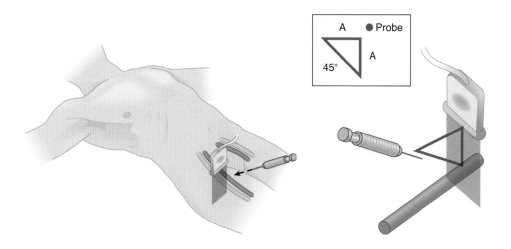

Tricks of the Trade

- The walls of the vein may tent inward when the needle approaches the vein. Extreme tenting (i.e., low vascular volume) may result in complete penetration of the anterior and posterior vein wall.

- Redirecting the needle once inside the patient during a difficult line placement will most likely result in no ultrasound guidance of the procedure. If the first pass is unsuccessful then remove needle from patient and start again from the beginning.

- Small rapid in-line movements of the needle (i.e., jiggling) during line placement will locate the needle tip on the screen by transmitting these movements to surrounding tissue.

- Veins become noncompressible when a clot is contained within their lumen. Always confirm patency of the vein by compressing it prior to cannulation attempt. If not compressible, consider using the contralateral side.

Still Image Protocol

Approach – Transverse plane, anterior
    Transducer at thigh
    Caudal to inguinal ligament
    Indicator toward right side
    Probe perpendicular to skin
    Image vein prior to
    introduction
      of needle
    Image vein during
    introduction
      of needle

Videotape Protocol

Video documentation of ultrasound uses the same landmarks and positioning as stills, but video allows for a dynamic documentation of the introduction of the needle into the vein. There is no movement of probe during procedure.

Ultrasound Guided Fluid Drainage

J. Christian Fox and Romolo Gaspari

Ultrasound Guided Thoracentesis

GOAL OF ULTRASOUND GUIDED THORACENTESIS

Facilitate draining fluid collections in the chest.

RATIONALE FOR ULTRASOUND GUIDED THORACENTESIS

Using ultrasound allows you to avoid puncturing the lung or liver by localizing an area of maximal fluid collection. If loculations are encountered, selective aspiration can be accomplished under real-time guidance.

ANATOMY

- Rib
- Scapula
- Liver
- Spleen
- Diaphragm
- Lung
- Intercostal muscles
- Clavicle

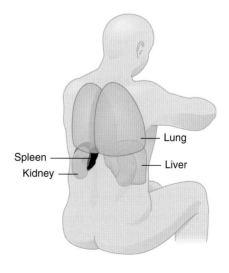

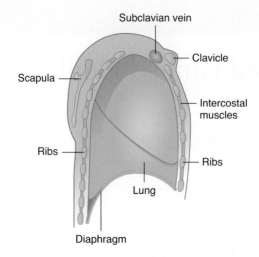

Note: Organs of the abdomen move cranially and caudally with expiration and inspiration, respectively, as the diaphragm contracts and relaxes. At full expiration the liver and spleen can be as high at the 10th thoracic rib.

PATIENT POSITION

- Sitting (preferred)
- Leaning forward

PATIENT PREPARATION

- Clean and disinfect skin

TRANSDUCER

- High-frequency linear probe
- Micro-convex curved probe (3–5 MHz)
          or
- Phased array probe
          or
- Linear probe (5–7 MHz)

ULTRASOUND IMAGE ELEMENTS

- Ribs
- Lung edge (pleura)
- Diaphragm (if inferior)
- Liver (if right side inferior)
- Spleen (if left side inferior)

Ultrasound Appearance of Fluid in the Thorax

- Free fluid in the chest should accumulate in a dependent area
- Loculated fluid in the chest may accumulate in pockets at any location

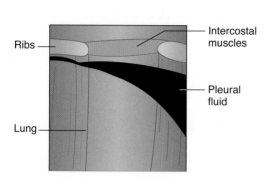

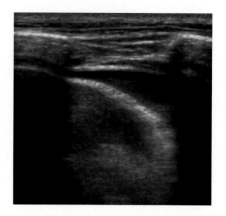

ULTRASOUND TECHNIQUE

- Position probe on lower, posterior chest wall
- Indicator to patient's head
- Locate largest fluid collection
- Identify superior border of fluid collection
- Identify rib space where needle will be inserted
- Image at point of needle insertion through multiple inspiratory and expiratory cycles to identify movement of internal organs

Procedure Technique

Still guidance
- Identify fluid collection
- Map superior border of fluid collection
- Identify location for needle insertion
  - Over largest pocket of fluid
  - Avoid internal organs (at full expiration)
  - Avoid neurovascular bundles under rib
- Remove probe and disinfect skin
- Anesthetize skin surface
- Insert needle at predetermined spot on chest wall

Dynamic guidance
- Disinfect skin surface
- Place probe in sterile cover
- Identify fluid collection
- Map superior border of fluid collection
- Identify location for needle insertion
  - Over largest pocket of fluid
  - Avoid internal organs (at full expiration)
  - Avoid neurovascular bundles under rib
- Anesthetize skin surface
- Insert needle next to probe head at exact center of probe, angled toward fluid
- Once fluid begins to flow into the syringe, the probe is securely placed aside and the procedure continues in the usual fashion.

The hyperechoic ring down artifact represents the metallic needle. Lung is seen as a hyperechoic homogenous structure containing occasional air shadows. It moves in and out as the patient breathes.

Tricks of the Trade

- In cases in which loculations are present, the probe can be continued to be used in order to guide the needle to the various loculations while taking care to avoid the lung.

- Dynamic guidance during a thoracentesis increases procedural complexity. Static guidance is usually adequate.

- Rotating probe may provide better imaging between ribs, but may make real-time guidance more challenging.

Still Image Protocol

Approach – Longitudinal plane, anterior
Transducer at lower posterior thorax
Indicator toward head
Probe perpendicular to skin
Angle and sweep stationary probe if needed to better visualize fluid
Image fluid collection prior to introduction of needle
Image needle entering fluid collection

Videotape Protocol

Video documentation of ultrasound uses the same landmarks and positioning as stills, but video allows for a dynamic documentation of the introduction of the needle into the fluid collection. There is no movement of probe during procedure.

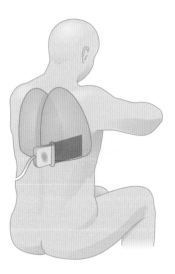
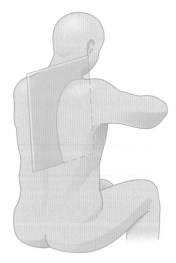

Ultrasound Guided Paracentesis
GOAL OF ULTRASOUND GUIDED PARACENTESIS

Facilitate draining fluid collections in the abdomen

RATIONALE FOR ULTRASOUND GUIDED PARACENTESIS

Using ultrasound allows you to avoid puncturing internal organs by localizing an area of maximal fluid collection. It increases the chances of a successful drainage when a small amount of fluid is present.

ANATOMY

- Liver
- Spleen
- Small bowel
- Large bowel
- Bladder
- Inferior epigastric artery

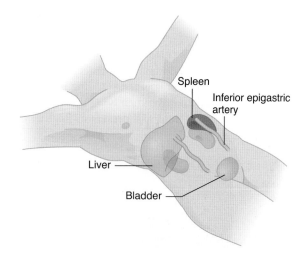

Note: The umbilicus marks the center of the abdomen. The needle should be introduced inferior or lateral to the umbilicus. Be sure to avoid the bladder (inferior) and inferior epigastric vasculature (lateral).

PATIENT POSITION

- Supine
- Lateral decub

PATIENT PREPARATION

- Clean and disinfect skin

TRANSDUCER

- Curved probe (3–5 MHz)
- Linear probe (5–10 MHz)

ULTRASOUND IMAGE ELEMENTS

- Abdominal wall
- Bowel loops
- Free fluid
- Needle

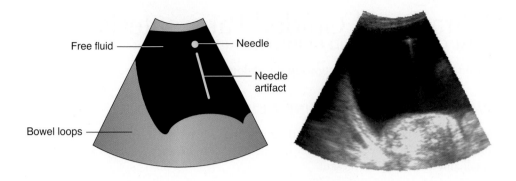

Ultrasound Appearance of Free Fluid in the Abdomen

- Free fluid will present as anechoic shapes with sharp angles
- Fluid in structures (bladder and bowel) will present as anechoic rounded shapes
- Free fluid in the abdomen should accumulate in dependent areas
  - Most dependent area when standing is the pelvis
  - Most dependent area when lying down is Morison's pouch
- Large amounts of fluid will present as floating bowel loops

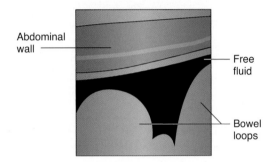

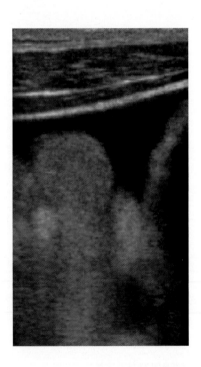

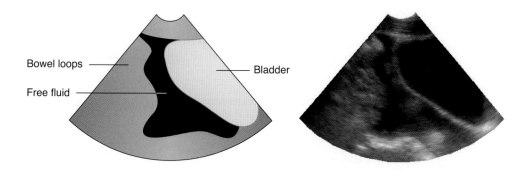

Bowel loops

Free fluid

Bladder

ULTRASOUND TECHNIQUE

- Position probe on anterior abdominal wall
- Indicator orientation is variable
- Locate largest fluid collection
- Identify structures bordering fluid collection

    The hyperechoic ring down artifact represents the metallic needle. Bowel gas presents as hazy linear shadows extending away from probe.

Procedure Technique

Still guidance
- Identify fluid collections
- Delineate borders of fluid collection
- Identify location for needle insertion
- Remove probe and disinfect skin
- Anesthetize skin surface
- Insert needle at predetermined spot on abdominal wall

Dynamic guidance
- Disinfect skin surface
- Place probe in sterile cover
- Identify fluid collection
- Delineate borders of fluid collection
- Identify location for needle insertion
- Anesthetize skin surface
- Insert needle next to probe head at center of probe, angled toward fluid
- Once fluid begins to flow into the syringe, the probe is placed aside and the procedure continues in the usual fashion

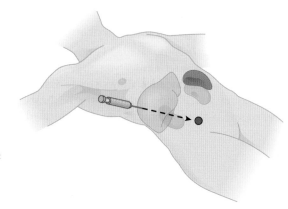

Tricks of the Trade

- Avoid inserting needle too inferiorly and therefore risk puncturing the bladder.

- Many patients with ascites have hepatosplenomegaly. Avoid inserting needle too superiorly as this can lead to liver and spleen punctures.

- Placing patient in lateral decubitus or reverse Trendelenburg may concentrate fluid and enable a successful procedure.

- In cases in which loculations are present, the probe can be continued to be used in order to guide the needle to the various loculations while taking care to avoid bowel, bladder, liver, and spleen.

- Identify structures between probe and fluid to prevent complications during needle insertion.

- Continued ultrasound during the fluid drainage may identify occlusion of catheter tip by bowel loops.

Still Image Protocol

Approach – Anterior abdomen
    Transducer inferior and lateral to umbilicus
    Indicator direction variable
    Probe perpendicular to skin
    Locate probe over fluid collection
    Image fluid collection prior to introduction of needle
    Image needle entering fluid collection

Videotape Protocol

Video documentation of ultrasound uses the same landmarks and positioning as stills, but video allows for a dynamic documentation of the introduction of the needle into the fluid collection. There is no movement of probe during procedure.

ULTRASOUND GUIDED PERICARDIOCENTESIS

Goal of Ultrasound Guided Pericardiocentesis

Facilitate draining fluid in the pericardium around the heart

Rationale for Ultrasound Guided Pericardiocentesis
    Using ultrasound allows you to visualize fluid collections in the pericardium. Using ultrasound guidance allows you to visualize introduction of the needle into the pericardium and avoid contact with the heart. Ultrasound guidance is not always needed and pericardiocentesis can be performed 'blind'.

ANATOMY

- Heart
- Diaphragm
- Liver
- Pericardial space

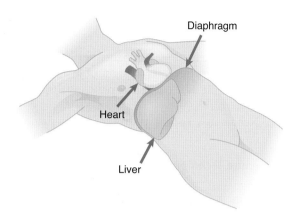

PATIENT POSITION

- Supine

Most pericardiocentesis performed in the emergency department are in patients with decreasing or unstable clinical status and are performed in a supine position.

PATIENT PREPARATION

- Clean and disinfect skin

TRANSDUCER

- Curved probe (3–5 MHz)
- Phased array probe (2–4 MHz)

ULTRASOUND IMAGE ELEMENTS

- Liver
- Cardiac Silouette
- Pericardial Space
- Needle

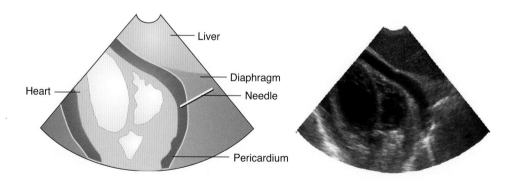

Ultrasound Appearance of Pericardial Effusion

- Free fluid around the heart will appear as an anechoic rim
- Pericardial fat pads can appear as a hypoechoic area next to the heart
  - Note – pericardial fat does not commonly surround the heart

Ultrasound Technique

- Position probe sub-costal
- Indicator orientation is to patient's right
- Position heart in center or right of image
- Image needle as it enters the pericardial space

Needle may appear as distinct linear shape or indistinct hyperechoic object with ring down artifact. Ring down artifact is repeating linear echoes posterior to needle.

Procedure Technique

Still Guidance
- Identify fluid collections
- Delineate extent of pericardial effusion
- Identify location for needle insertion
- Remove probe and disinfect skin (if time permits)
- Insert needle at pre-determined spot on abdominal wall in direction of heart

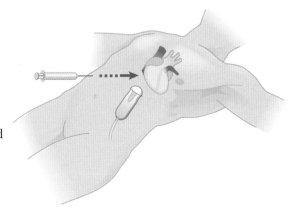

Dynamic Guidance
- Disinfect skin surface
- Place probe in sterile cover
- Identify fluid collection
- Delineate extent of pericardial effusion
- Identify location for needle insertion
- Insert needle in epigastrium angling towards heart
- Maneuver probe to image needle entering pericardium
- Once fluid begins to flow into the syringe, the probe is placed aside and the procedure continues in the usual fashion

---

Tricks of the Trade

- Pericardial fat pads can mimic effusions
  - Fat pads are not circumferential
  - Diameter of fat pad does not change as heart beats
  - There are usually echoes in fat pads

- If the epigastrim is too crowded, move the ultrasound probe and image from left or right sub-costal.

Still Image Protocol

Approach – Anterior Abdomen
    Transducer inferior to xyphoid process
    Indicator direction to patient's right
    Probe at shallow angle to abdominal wall
    Locate heart in center of screen
    Image pericardial fluid collection prior to introduction of needle
    Image needle entering pericardium

Video Tape Protocol

Video documentation of ultrasound uses the same landmarks and positioning as stills, but video allows for a dynamic documentation of the introduction of the needle into the fluid collection. There is no movement of probe during procedure. Ultrasound may offer additional information on cardiac performance following procedure.

Using Type Projects